Young People and the Aesthetics of Health Promotion

Health promotion with young people has largely been framed by theories of behaviour change to target 'unsafe', 'unhealthy' and/or 'risky' behaviours. These theories and models seek to encourage the development in young people of reasoned, rational and risk-aware personal strategies.

This book presents an innovative and critical perspective on young people and health promotion. It explores the limits and possibilities of traditional health behaviour change models with their focus on reason, risk and rationality by examining the embodied dimensions of meaning-making in health promotion programs. Drawing on an array of critical social theories and approaches to knowledge production, the authors identify and engage the aesthetic and affective dimensions of young people's engagement with issues such as road safety, sexualities, alcohol and drug use, and physical and mental health and well-being.

The book will appeal to researchers and practitioners in the fields of health promotion and health education, public health, education, the sociology of health and illness, youth studies and youth work.

Kerry Montero is Program Manager of the Bachelor of Social Science Youth Work program at RMIT University, Melbourne, Australia.

Peter Kelly is Deputy Head of School (Research and Innovation) and Director, Centre for Education, Training and Work in the Asian Century, in the School of Education, RMIT University.

Youth, Young Adulthood and Society

Series editor: Andy Furlong, University of Glasgow, UK | Andy.Furlong@glasgow.ac.uk

The **Youth, Young Adulthood and Society** series brings together social scientists from many disciplines to present research monographs and collections, seeking to further research into youth in our changing societies around the world today. The books in this series advance the field of youth studies by presenting original, exciting research, with strongly theoretically and empirically grounded analysis.

Published:

Body Work
Youth, Gender and Health
Julia Coffey

Young People and the Aesthetics of Health Promotion
Beyond Reason, Rationality and Risk
Kerry Montero and Peter Kelly

The Subcultural Imagination
Theory, Research and Reflexivity in Contemporary Youth Cultures
Edited by Shane Blackman and Michelle Kempson

Forthcoming:

Young People in the Labour Market
Past, Present, Future
Andy Furlong, John Goodwin, Sarah Hadfield, Stuart Hall, Kevin Lowden and Henrietta O'Connor

Youth, Class and Culture
Steven Threadgold

Spaces of Youth
Identities, Inequalities and Social Change
David Farrugia

Rethinking Young People's Marginalisation
Beyond Neo-Liberal Futures?
Perri Campbell, Lyn Harrison, Chris Hickey and Peter Kelly

Muslim Youth in the Diaspora
Challenging Extremism through Popular Culture
Pam Nilan

Young People and the Aesthetics of Health Promotion

Beyond reason, rationality and risk

Kerry Montero and Peter Kelly

Routledge
Taylor & Francis Group
LONDON AND NEW YORK

First published 2016
by Routledge

2 Park Square, Milton Park, Abingdon, Oxfordshire OX14 4RN
52 Vanderbilt Avenue, New York, NY 10017

Routledge is an imprint of the Taylor & Francis Group, an informa business

First issued in paperback 2019

British Library Cataloguing in Publication Data
A catalogue record for this book is available from the British Library

Library of Congress Cataloging in Publication Data
Names: Montero, Kerry, author. | Kelly, Peter, 1957- author.
Title: Young people and the aesthetics of health promotion : beyond reason, rationality and risk / Kerry Montero and Peter Kelly.
Description: Milton Park, Abingdon, Oxon ; New York, NY : Routledge, 2016. |
Series: Youth, young adulthood and society
Identifiers: LCCN 2015040288| ISBN 9781138898059 (hbk) |
ISBN 9781315708805 (ebk)
Subjects: LCSH: Health promotion. | Health education. | Health behavior in adolescence. | Young adults--Health aspects.
Classification: LCC RA427.8 .M66 2016 | DDC 613/.0433--dc23
LC record available at http://lccn.loc.gov/2015040288

ISBN: 978-1-138-89805-9 (hbk)
ISBN: 978-0-367-35293-6 (pbk)

Typeset in Times New Roman
by Taylor & Francis Books

Kerry. For Ruben, Nina, Ben and Daniel
Peter. For Georgia

Contents

List of boxes ix
Prelude x

Introduction **1**
Health promotion as a complex assemblage 1
Fit to Drive, young people, and embodied health promotion 8
Embodiment and the aesthetics of meaning making 12
Structure of the book 14

1 School based health promotion as a complex assemblage **20**
In the beginning … 20
The 'irreal' spaces of schools 24
'Take any empty space …': transforming the space, becoming theatre 29
The players in a school based performance 33
Mobilising for the good? 37

2 Rationality and risk: Limits and possibilities **41**
Breath *and the horror of the mundane 41*
'Cold, hard facts' 44
Young people and road safety: a health promotion problem made known through risk 47
Young people and the problem of risk 52
Beyond rationality and risk? 60

3 Engaging emotions, exploring values, mobilising rationality **64**
'A moment of emotional truth …' 64
Health education, youth work and values 69
Rediscovering emotions 77
Health promotion and emotion as 'embodied sociality' 81

4 'Do, then talk': Young people, group work and the making of meaning **85**
Does her body think? 85
Embodied meaning making 87
Do … 90
… then talk 95
Body and language: partners in a conversation 98

5 'What happened was this … ': What roles do stories have in health promotion? **103**
Birthday *and 'Shannon's Story' 105*
'Graham's Story' and the 'ur-' stories in Fit to Drive 107
Storytelling, audience and narrative devices 108
The characteristics of story and narrative: lessons for health promotion 113
Story, empathy and understanding 118
Narrative quest and the pursuit of the moral in health promotion 121

6 A Greek tragedy: Chaos and control **125**
The Monavale tragedy 125
'It's just one of those things that's all gone wrong': fear and pity and the Monavale story as tragedy 131
The tragedy goes to work: Brandon Glen Secondary College, November 2009 136
The tragic and the problem of death 138

7 Young people as choosing agents? **145**
The dangerousness of risk 145
Talking about and rating the risks 149
'Stop the car! I'm going to be sick!' 155
Beyond agency in health promotion with young people? 163

Conclusion **171**
Death and devastation as allegory 171
Reordering health promotion with young people 174

References 180
Index 194

Boxes

Interlude: Kerry's story xi
Interlude: the aesthetics and erotics of the human-car-machine assemblage 56
Interlude: Brecht and the 'theatre of emotions' 74
Interlude: 'Fridays with Graham', November 2009. Talking about feelings, behaviours, consequences 79
Kerry's story: understanding Jim 118
Kerry's story: Aeschylus or Aesop? 130
Interlude: Kerry's story 178

Prelude

A single line from a 2009 news story titled 'Seven Teens in Horrific Car Crash' describes a stark scenario that would be all too familiar for too many people in too many cities and communities in too many countries around the globe.

> A split-second decision to overload a car has left two teenagers dead and three others fighting for their lives.
>
> (Burley 2009)

The news report describing the barest details of a crash that occurred on a Saturday night in rural Australia is just the beginning of a story that will unfold in layer upon layer of grief, recriminations, questioning and guilt, as the events of this night are played and replayed for years, decades to come. They will affect the lives of untold numbers of people beyond the epicentre of the event, and will involve spin-off events and processes – police charges, court cases and enquiries, public responses – that will make those involved relive the trauma again and again. The regional police inspector who is interviewed for the story is acutely aware of the 'far-reaching effects' of the tragedy:

> 'In a place like Toowoomba, everyone will know someone affected by this tragedy,' he said. 'It will ripple through the entire community.'

As we read the news story we play it in our minds, imagining, and empathising. Will the young men survive? What will their lives look like? How will their parents cope? And so the story will be played forwards, and possible futures imagined and mapped. But it will be played backwards as well. How is it that so many young men – just 16 and 17 years old, at the threshold of life – were in the one car? Why were they in the boot? Didn't they realise the danger? And, crucially, what could we have done to prevent this?

In any given week we could retrieve a similar report that would describe a version of a similar story. Road crashes involving young people occur with disheartening regularity world-wide. Despite significant road toll reductions in

Australia since 1990, young drivers continue to have more casualty crashes than any other group of drivers on the road. While making up less than 15 per cent of all licensed drivers, people aged 18–25 account for 28 per cent of driver deaths (TAC 2012), and crash risk in the first year of driving is more than three times greater than in subsequent years (Healy et al. 2012). In 2003 in Victoria (Australia) nearly fifty young drivers were killed, 100 young people were involved in fatal crashes, and 7,000 were in casualty crashes (MacKenzie 2003). Although the number of young drivers killed has been reduced since 2003, road crashes remain one of the biggest killers of young people aged 16–25 in Victoria and Australia (Eldridge 2008; AIHW 2011).

This sort of news story speaks to a range of emotions such as grief, rage, futility and the helplessness set loose by the reality of death and injury of young people on our roads. This book, in part, focuses on a particular effort to intervene in this relentless repetition of road crashes involving young people. Part of our focus is on a school based road safety program, 'Fit to Drive', that had its beginnings in a small school community reeling from the loss of seven young lives within a period of 18 months. The program evolved as an expression of people's need to make sense of events that, seemingly randomly, had upended their world and shaken their faith in an ordered, predictable cosmos. Road trauma prevention is, ultimately, an attempt to reclaim order out of chaos, to assert control over the circumstances that lead to injury and death for too many young people. In the case of those involved in developing Fit to Drive, it required a journey of learning – about road safety, about the location and use of available resources and strategies, and the opportunities for road safety education offered by the school environment – and the search for the most effective way to integrate these elements to connect with and engage the creative energy of young people to find solutions to road trauma among their peers.

Interlude: Kerry's story[1]

Fit to Drive, for me, and for others who were there 'in the beginning', is identifiable through specific times and places: meeting the Young Driver Committee at Karingal Secondary College; meetings over coffee at Druids café (a familiar RMIT University city haunt); the first facilitator training session at Mt Erin Secondary College; the launch and first school workshop. It is a history that has key turning points, serendipitous meetings of people and events and moments of reflection, analysis and insight.

The character of Fit to Drive – the educational philosophy, the community orientation, the promotion of young peoples' voice – reflects the combined interests and experience of former school principal Graham Spencer, Bern Rowland-Ariens (a youth work graduate and trained teacher) and myself as we met and developed the workshop idea, then the broader program. It became refined and embedded through the training of facilitators and workshop debriefs, through write-up of the program documentation, and through the process of preparing for conferences and presentations.

My reflections on Fit to Drive (the way it works, what it does) take me to the beginnings of the program's development.

As I think about how I will write about Fit to Drive I gradually come to realise that I will need to place myself within the story. In this positioning we can learn some lessons from poststructuralism, which 'directs us to understand ourselves reflexively, as persons writing from *particular positions at specific times*' (Richardson 1998, p. 349, emphasis added). In this sense: 'Narratives about contexts in which the writing is produced ... evoke new questions about the self and the subject; they remind us that our work is grounded, contextual, and rhizomatic' (Richardson 2000, p. 931).

From the 1970s, in Australia, and particularly in Victoria, diverse policies and programs had made a major impact on the high rate of road fatalities by introducing a series of legislative initiatives, including compulsory seatbelt legislation, alcohol restrictions, speed detection and enforcement. At the same time a significant concern was the continued over-representation of young people in road crashes. (Cavallo and Triggs 1996). In the mid-1990s VicRoads, the road transport authority in the state of Victoria, had begun to turn its attention to the specific problem of young driver safety.

The responses to young people's over-representation in road crashes have been partly legislative, partly educational. Early efforts to reduce road trauma focused, from the early 1970s, on universal, largely engineering-based approaches: road design, vehicle design, seat-belt legislation. Alcohol restrictions and speed regulation targeted obvious problem behaviours. These measures saw a dramatic decrease in the number of road deaths, from more than 1,000 in Victoria in 1970 to around 340 by the early 1990s (Cavallo 2004). Over the past decade, as road trauma statistics have declined, but the continued over-representation of young people in these statistics has created cause for concern, many road safety interventions have focused specifically on young drivers. Recent initiatives to increase regulation of young drivers include graduated licensing, extension of the supervised learning period, broadening of restrictions on mobile phone use and the number of passengers young people can drive with, the horse-power limits of the cars young people can drive, and so-called 'anti-hoon' legislation that can confiscate the cars of young people who are convicted of reckless or dangerous driving (VicRoads 2005; Healy et al. 2012).

Road safety authorities – VicRoads, the Transport Accident Commission (TAC), the Department of Education and Early Childhood Development (DEECD) Traffic Safety Education Unit, the Victoria Police – have developed educational interventions aiming to change behaviours that are understood to put young people at risk on the roads. Initially attention was focused on the small but significant group of very high-risk young people, with specific interventions targeting extremely high risks, such as car theft, illegal racing, and unlicensed driving. Since then initiatives have been developed which argue for the universal risks associated with driving for all young people. These initiatives focus on inexperience as the single most significant causal factor in road crashes amongst young people. In addition, these interventions target the key factors associated with crash risk – speed, alcohol and other drugs, fatigue, distractions (VicRoads 2005). In this context VicRoads decided to explore the potential role of youth workers in the education of the cohort of 'hard to reach', 'at-risk' young people, who were identified as comprising the difficult end of the crash risk spectrum (Cavallo 1994). Youth workers, already engaged in personal and social skill development group programs and, to a certain degree, health education and health promotion, were well positioned to incorporate road safety education and awareness into their work (Batsleer 2008; Payne 2005). Initial research indicated that youth workers were identifying road safety issues and high-risk driving behaviours among their client group and there would be justification in developing resources, training and programs for youth workers to deliver road safety education and awareness to young people (Maunders and Sangster 1995; Cavallo et al. 1997). Working in the Bachelor of Arts (Youth Affairs) program at RMIT University, and with a background in health education, I was invited to participate in the development of road safety programs in youth work settings. This work resulted in the final version of the road safety program being published as 'Survival on the Roads' which was accompanied by a series of training workshops for workers (Montero et al. 1997). Subsequently a follow-up program was developed for newly licensed young drivers, 'Reducing the Toll' (Montero et al. 2002). I also became involved in the development of local government strategy for young drivers (Montero 2002).

I had been working in young road-user safety for over five years when I was put in contact with the group of schools and community organisations that had formed a committee to tackle the high rate of road trauma among young people on the Mornington Peninsula, southeast of Melbourne. In 2000 and 2001 there had been a spate of serious crashes that had involved young people who attended a number of the schools in the area. In a period of eighteen months, seven young people lost their lives in that region, leaving others injured, and the whole school community deeply impacted by these deaths. This led to the formation of the Frankston-Mornington Peninsula Young Driver Safety committee. When I first encountered them this committee was at the stage of looking for effective, viable traffic safety initiatives. They had organised a public 'fun-run' as a way of raising community awareness about the issue, and funds for educational programs about young driver safety. They had named the local initiative 'Fit to Drive'.

It is understandable that, when confronted by the terrible reality of the immense sadness, upheaval and questioning that follows a fatal car crash, we will search for unequivocal causes, reducible to clear, simple solutions. Sometimes there is a relatively clear and direct match between cause and event, and cause and solution. In many instances there is an apparent, clearly defined link (young people and high crash rates) but no one obvious cause. Young driver research shows a link between crashes and such things as: when young people drive (night time); who they drive with (young friends or parents); what they've been doing (drinking or taking drugs, studying all night for exams) (Harrison 2006; Williams 2003). Such findings affirm common sense intuitions and understandings of the problem.

A magic formula, a clearly delineated solution, didn't exist for the community on the Mornington Peninsula when they were galvanised into action. They had to search out their own, acknowledging that there is no 'one solution' to the problem of road trauma, and that any initiative would need to be long term, based on evidence and good practice. VicRoads' representatives on the Frankston-Mornington Peninsula Committee suggested the resources and examples of good practice represented by 'Survival on the Roads' and 'Reducing the Toll' would be useful to draw on in developing ideas for interventions. Initial discussion with the committee – consisting mainly of principals of participating schools, with local government roads safety officers and VicRoads representatives – led to the idea of an education workshop for senior students, bringing together organisations working in road safety education, who, it was claimed, had traditionally worked in an uncoordinated, fragmented way.

Fit to Drive was, then, initially developed as a road safety program for students in years 10, 11 and 12 of secondary school. As it developed it was distinguished by the way it has been able to coordinate the activities, programs and resources developed by road safety stakeholders for young people (including VicRoads, the Transport Accident Commission, Victoria Police and the Metropolitan Fire Brigade). The cornerstone of the program is a half-day workshop for year 11 students which features presentations by road safety education agencies and small group discussion workshops facilitated by trained tertiary students from youth work, social work and education programs. The students, 'near peer' in age, are explicitly named as road safety role models, or 'ambassadors', a recognition of their potential for positive influence on the secondary students in relation to responsible driving and passenger behaviour. Through a variety of activities the workshops provide the opportunity for senior secondary students to explore and challenge their attitudes and beliefs in relation to driving, relate their own experiences, undertake problem-solving and decision-making exercises in relation to driving situations and support their peers in adopting safer practices. The program's aims are to 'support young people to make positive choices in relation to driving and road use' by 'raising awareness (in young people) of the risks and factors that contribute to road crashes in their age group', and using peer education strategies to develop capacities to 'avoid crashes and resist peer pressure influences' (Spencer et al. 2006, p. 6). The program reinforces the need for young drivers to obtain 120 hours of supervised on-road practice in all types of driving conditions in order to lessen the effect of inexperience as a factor in road crashes. A significant feature of the entire program is that young people work with their peers to identify strategies to reduce high-risk situations, and to identify school and community initiatives to promote road safety in their local area.

And so Fit to Drive was developed, with a central guiding principle that it would be as much about listening to young people's experience and views on road safety, and engaging them in solutions, as providing information and safe messages. The program has been developed and refined since then, during which time it has been conducted each year in every secondary school on the Frankston-Mornington Peninsula, as well as a growing number of school regions throughout Melbourne and the state of Victoria such as Greater Dandenong, Macedon Ranges, Geelong and Bendigo. By 2010 Fit to Drive had grown from an initial eighteen schools in the one region to approximately 160 across ten metropolitan and country regions (Spencer and Montero 2011).

In this book we are interested, then, in exploring the 'meeting-places' where certain ideas and representations about young people, risk and road safety as a problem are presented, invoked – their authority enacted – at various levels and in different forms. We want to explore how these ideas meet, connect and interact with the understandings, experience and 'being-in-the-world' of the young people in the space of the Fit to Drive workshop, and how the young people receive the messages – intentional, unintentional, contradictory and consistent – that are transmitted in the context of the program. To do this we draw out the meanings derived from the stories and interactions, the meetings with peers and facilitators and presenters; the world the young people inhabit as they engage in meaning making. We put into play personal experiences during a long engagement with the program (Kerry's stories); we mobilise video/audio recorded data from the workshops, observations, reflections and field notes. In the background, sometimes the foreground, is our own history of collaboration and conversation that in an embodied sense began with the Ph.D. student–supervisor relationship, but continues, now, to draw on engagements with the written word, the published work of both of us.

So this book, like all books, is an embodied enactment of meaningmaking. And for this book to make sense in the terms we set for it we need some techniques to make these embodied enactments present on the page. At various times, then, the reader will encounter 'Interludes', asides where background thinking, something that in other contexts would remain 'manifestly absent', or 'absent as Other' (Law 2004), is made present. At other times fragments of 'Kerry's Story' (presented as 'Interludes') are used to embody meaning making because other means available to us don't work in those spaces. While the focus in much of the discussion is on Fit to Drive, and how we might understand the aesthetic dimensions of meaning making on/at the limits of reason, risk and rationality, we will argue that there are wider lessons about the limits and possibilities of aesthetics, reason, risk and rationality for an array of school based health promotion interventions that target young people. Our hope is that these lessons, this meaning making, will become clearer at different times in what follows.

Note

1 Later we will provide a brief account of some of the fieldwork based research from which this book, in part, emerges, and the roles that 'Kerry's Story', as an 'Interlude', will play throughout this discussion.

Introduction

Health promotion as a complex assemblage

At the beginning of his *After Method*, John Law (2004, p. 1) references the White Queen from Lewis Carroll's *Through the Looking Glass*, and her fantastical claim to believe in *impossible things*:

> 'There's no use in trying,' [Alice said]: 'one can't believe impossible things.' 'I daresay you haven't had much practice,' said the Queen. 'When I was your age, I always did it for half-an-hour a day. Why, sometimes I've believed as many as six impossible things before breakfast.'

Over a number of years Law (2004) has made a provocative contribution to ongoing discussions about what he and Annemarie Mol (Mol and Law 2006) identify as knowledge practices in the social and the hard sciences. Law's work is most often associated with studies of Science, Technology and Society (STS), actor-network theory and a more generalised interest in complexities, heterogeneities and knowledge practices in the natural and social sciences. In *After Method* Law (2004) makes reference to a wider intellectual debt to the challenges and possibilities posed by feminism and post-structuralism to disciplines such as sociology. At the same time he firmly locates his project in STS. Law stresses that traditional scientific (social, hard) knowledge practices craft realities that, in many instances, produce knowledge, outcomes and consequences that have been, are, important. However, if, as Law (2004, p. 2) suggests, so much of the natural, the social and the cultural is 'vague, diffuse or unspecific, slippery, emotional, ephemeral, elusive or indistinct', then can the institutionalised, even standardised, rule-bound knowledge practices of the social sciences – quantitative and/or qualitative methods such as interviews, surveys, observations; forms of representation such as reports, theses, papers, monographs; practices such as interventions, programs, reviews, audits – capture or create understandings that can account for these realities? Or, do we need to 'teach ourselves to know some of the realities of the world using methods unusual to or unknown in social science'?

In exploring the limits and possibilities of standardised, orthodox method assemblages (knowledge practices) Law (2004, pp. 2–4) introduces and develops a vocabulary to shape the ways in which the social sciences might *think* and *know* differently (a number of these draw on feminist and post-structuralist discourses). For example, he discusses knowing as embodiment, where we come to know 'through the hungers, tastes, discomfort, or pains of our bodies'. Knowing as 'emotionality or apprehension' suggests, for Law, exploring 'private emotions' that bring into view the 'worlds of sensibilities, passions, intuitions, fears and betrayals'. Echoing feminist unsettling of discourses of objectivity and generalisability, Law proposes that we need to consider 'how far whatever it is that we know travels and whether it still makes sense in other locations and if so how. This would be knowing as situated inquiry'. In a final suggestion that points to allegory as a key motif in his discussions, Law argues that we need to think about and embrace the sense that our ways of knowing – despite our desires to dress them up in pretensions of validity, certainty and rigour – are, always, imprecise. In this sense we need to 'find ways of knowing the indistinct and the slippery without trying to grasp and hold them tight. Here knowing would become possible through techniques of deliberate imprecision' (see, also, Kelly 2011).

Law's work is not unique, but as we have argued elsewhere (Kelly 2013, 2012, 2011), it does provide a generative vocabulary for capturing and locating much of what interests us as we introduce and engage with the limits and possibilities of reason, risk, rationality and aesthetics in health promotion interventions that target young people, and the forms of description, analysis and critique that are able to explore and make sense of these limits and possibilities. A central, productive and generative idea that Law develops and introduces to this vocabulary is his notion, drawing on the different but related work of Gilles Deleuze and Bruno Latour, of *method assemblage*. For Law (2004, p. 144), method assemblage suggests a 'continuing process of crafting and enacting necessary boundaries' between 'presence, manifest absence, and absence as Otherness'. Any method/methodology/assemblage 'makes something present by making absence'. Method assemblage, in playing with the relations between presence, manifest absence and absence as Otherness, tries to make explicit and imagine the consequences of the 'crafting, bundling, or gathering of relations' between these elements. Between what Law identifies as 'in-here or present (for instance a representation or an object)'; between what is 'absent but also manifest (it can be seen, is described, is manifestly relevant to presence)', and, finally, between what is 'absent but is Other because, while necessary to presence, it is also hidden, repressed or uninteresting'. That which is Other:

> might range from things that everyone in question knows (how to do chromatography), through mundanities that no one notices until they stop happening (the supply of electricity), to matters or processes that are actively suppressed in order to produce the representations that are taken

> to report directly on realities (these would include the active character of authorship or the trail of continuities between statements and the realities that they describe).
>
> (Law 2004, p. 42)

Social science emerges from institutionalised spaces that demand particular approaches to knowledge production. These demands are not necessarily bad, as Foucault (1983) might say, but they do place limits on the ways, the methods that are considered appropriate for producing knowledge that is understood as useful. In these domains some can speak and others can't. Some things can be said and done and others can't. Certain ideas, stories, ways of producing knowledge are just impossible to imagine as being useful, appropriate, truthful, evidence based. And where useful signals something that is readily translatable, transferable, able to be operationalised by various agencies, departments, organisations in settings, processes and practices that may be remote and abstracted from the times/spaces/places where knowledge is produced. The tensions and dilemmas we see here relate to what those things that are absent, Othered, impossible might contribute to our understanding if they could be imagined as possible. Because, as Law (2004, p. 92) argues, in our everyday, sense-making existence we are all – expert and non-expert, scientist and artist – 'allegorists'. We 'read between the lines and manifest realities that are not being spoken about in as many words'. We unsettle, interfere with the 'boundaries between that which is Othered and that which is manifest'. In this way we can imagine allegory as a 'mode of discovery – so long as we understand that in a world of enactment, allegory is also crafting what it is discovering'. In addition, as allegorists we, much of the time, 'are crafting and manifesting realities that are non-coherent. That are difficult to fit together into a single smooth reality' (Kelly 2013, 2011).

This constant bundling, unravelling, fixing, troubling of the relationships between presence, manifest absence and absence as Otherness will be a key motif throughout much of this book. This vocabulary allows a particular approach to description, discussion, analysis and critique that opens up the shifting relationships between reason, risk, rationality and the embodied aesthetics of meaning making that we think are important in exploring and understanding the limits and possibilities of school based health promotion with young people. At different times this book engages with questions such as 'What can we know?' 'How can we know?' 'How do we construct that *knowing*?' All in relation to the 'problem' of young drivers and road safety. But more broadly we explore the limits and possibilities of mobilising ideas of aesthetics, reason, risk and rationality in the doing of school based health promotion with young people. The book's analysis explores the limits and possibilities of traditional health behaviour change models to examine the deeper dimensions of engagement and meaning making within health promotion programs. As we draw on detailed research conducted on Fit to Drive we will suggest key dimensions that have resonance and applicability in relation to other areas of health promotion, and social education, with young people.

Health promotion and education have traditionally tended to focus on the design of programs based on behaviour change theory to target 'unsafe', 'unhealthy' and/or 'risky' behaviours. We recognise and will acknowledge that behaviour change models such as participatory (peer-led) facilitated discussion, and the development of reasoned, rational and risk-aware personal strategies, resistance and assertiveness skills, are an integral part of the design of many health promotion interventions and programs. The contributions that we want to make to thinking about the array of health promotion programs that target young people will come from identifying, then exploring and analysing, the aesthetic dimensions of program design and delivery that create the possibilities for meaning making.

From a base where we review the existing and extensive multi-disciplinary (psychological, sociological, cultural studies) literature on health promotion with young people, we will draw on theoretical approaches from phenomenological and narrative research traditions, as well as, at different times, post-structuralist and governmentality studies, to develop an understanding of the elements that are essential to the character of the program that is experienced by participants. At different times through the book, and in different ways, we will provide an analysis of the individual elements and modes of engagement in the Fit to Drive program – the activities, the different modes of delivery, the role of stories, narratives, tragedy, emotion, reason, rationality and risk – to reveal the ways they work together in the context of the school setting to make something *meaningful.*

Our aim is to unsettle, to trouble, to make problematic approaches to understanding the factors and strategies that promise to provide successful health promotion interventions in the school, and in other health promotion settings. The strategies and approaches that emerge from this analysis – including a sense of health promotion as often tragic theatre, of the always embodied dimensions of meaning making, of the role of the 'audience', and the limits and possibilities of mobilising morally charged emotions and story-telling – offer innovative theoretical, methodological and empirical insights into the challenges of 'doing' and 'critiquing' health promotion *for* young people.

Any approach to an understanding of young people, driving and road safety, and to broader concerns about young people's physical and mental health and well-being, their sexualities and uses of alcohol and drugs, must journey along paths laid down by established disciplines that have mapped the terrain by means of statistical analysis, psychological investigations, socio-cultural studies, developmental theory and, more recently, the application of neuro-scientific theories of young people and risk-taking (see for example Jessor 1987; Mayhew et al. 2002; Peden et al. 2004; Toroyan and Peden 2007; Vassallo et al. 2007; Weiss 2006). Popular and 'serious' media also contribute to the creation of a strong culture of scrutiny and search for explanation/understanding of these problems (Begley 2000; Catalyst 2005; Reyna and

Farley 2007; Sabbagh 2006). Indeed, it could be argued that they play a central role in the 'problem-setting' (Bessant 2002) in relation to young people and concerns about their health and well-being.

Road safety research, for example, draws from many different fields to construct different knowledges in relation to road injury prevention: 'The public health approach to road safety is based on science. It draws on knowledge from medicine, biomechanics, epidemiology, sociology, behavioural science, criminology, education, economics, engineering and other disciplines' (Peden et al. 2004, p. 3). Engineering disciplines analyse road- and vehicle-related factors involved in crashes; epidemiological research investigates patterns of crashes and road user behaviour; 'human sciences' inform understandings of prevention and intervention, in the guise of education, health promotion approaches and law enforcement. Young driver research generally proceeds from an acknowledgement of the complexities inherent in understanding and explaining road crashes involving young drivers At the same time there is a history of difficulties in establishing dialogue between, for instance, engineering, law enforcement and educational approaches to road safety. Current public policy seeks to combine insights from the respective discipline areas to develop a response that is seen to be consistent with this research, and that addresses the complexities of the problem. With respect to young drivers, legislative measures such as the Graduated Licensing System have built on road safety research that demonstrates links between high crash rates and inexperience, as well as understandings of driving contexts and young driver characteristics that contribute to (or are implicated in) road crashes (Healy et al. 2012; Mayhew 2007; VicRoads 2005).

These, then, represent different – possibly complementary, sometimes conflicting – ways of 'knowing' the problem of young people and road crashes. Most of these explanatory approaches are aware of each other, and may nod, or even 'speak' to each other on some levels (Peden et al. 2004). Road safety public policy does recognise complexity, and acknowledges at some level the 'whole person' within the social context, built environment and realm of human action (Doherty et al. 1998). It does this by responding on several 'fronts', including through education, legislation in relation to licensing, law enforcement, and even early intervention with 'at risk' children and young people. However, neither public policy or road safety research acknowledges the social construction of problems: the problem of young drivers is taken as a given, evidenced by the statistical picture: 'The elevated crash risk of teenage drivers is well known' (Williams 2003, p. 5). From this perspective, the business of research is to describe the problem, clarify causes and contribute to the development of solutions. It assumes as 'natural' the category of 'young person' and ignores the political position/ing and economic experience of young people at different historical moments. Recent writings in critical youth studies complicate the dominant interpretations of young people and traffic safety. Some youth studies writers have called into question the construction of young people as specifically susceptible to higher crash involvement and have expressed reservations about the positioning of young people as requiring specific attention and interventions in relation to their status as drivers. The identification/construction of the 'young driver problem' has been linked to the established practice of the creation of conservative moral panics related to young people (Best 2008; Males 2006), and framed by the language of 'risk'. In these discourses young people are positioned as a problem and target for specialised, and sometimes problematic, interventions (Bessant et al. 2003; Kelly 1998, 2003). The introduction, in many jurisdictions, of Graduated Licensing Systems (GLS) for young drivers has been identified as a specific instance of such discriminatory practice (Best 2008; Males 2005).

In road safety research there is therefore a privileging of certain disciplines – epidemiology and other applications of statistical analysis, engineering, behavioural psychology, statistical sociology – as accepted 'ways of knowing' road safety. This mirrors the hegemony of certain (science-based) forms of knowledge and methods of inquiry in Euro-American research environments (see Law 2004 for a discussion of this; see also Denzin and Lincoln 2008; Flyvbjerg 2006; Gadamer 2006). Diverse areas of science writing have challenged the limited and inappropriate application of the methods and epistemological foundations of the natural sciences to the study of human behaviour and complex social and human phenomena (Gould 1981; Rose 2005). Tracing the genesis of this hierarchical division of knowledge/s in western intellectual inquiry, some authors emphasise the political and social foundations of this development. The disciplines themselves have been, as Elizabeth Grosz observes: 'effects of concrete, dynamic, historically and culturally specific relations of power' (Grosz 1995, p. 27).

Methods employed by natural and physical science disciplines are effective in explaining the physical world (Midgley 2003; Law 2004). Epidemiology has helped to discover important links between certain behaviours or phenomena and specific illnesses and diseases (Lupton and Petersen 1996). And social research methodologies that use quantitative methods and statistical analysis have been successful in demonstrating links between social inequalities and individual and social harms (Law 2004). They are not so successful, however, in explaining 'human experience of the world and human living' (Gadamer 2006, p. xxvii).

Significant aspects of road safety involve human behaviour, human subjectivity and inter-subjectivity, and are not amenable to reductionist explanations. Road safety is a good example of the need for approaches to 'knowing' a problem to proceed from an understanding of the way we 'share a world' – 'one world, but a big one' – in the sense described by Mary Midgley (2006). A single explanatory account won't give us a full insight into the 'reality' of young driver crashes. Explanations, as Midgley (2006, p. 170) observes, 'come in various kinds. They vary with the needs that call for them. "Explaining things" does not necessarily mean fitting them into existing scientific schemes. It means placing them on the wider map of our thought.'

From this perspective a consideration of young people's own capacities for meaning making and action should be central to any critique of contemporary young driver discourse, in which public policy and media representations are seen to frame young people as a 'problem' in relation to road safety. Young people's own understandings, their own stories, their engagement with the issue – which may include a deep personal connection with the experience of road trauma – are central to the ways young people position themselves in relation to road safety and risk. How should we understand the 'young driver problem' as a 'governmentalised' (institutionalised, rationalised and abstract) object (Kelly 2011), in the light of the experience, the reality of the stories that are told over and again by young people in the Fit to Drive workshops and facilitator training sessions? These stories tell of young people's own experience of losing brothers, sisters, friends. What do we make of the motivations of the young people who return to be trained as peer facilitators after experiencing the program as year 11 students a few years previously: often following the loss of fellow students to car crashes, and who had felt deeply affected and wanting to 'do' something?

Midgley's description of 'one world, but a big one' to illustrate the multiple possibilities of understanding and interpreting the world, is echoed in Law's (2004, p. 8) call to honour the richness of the world by recognising, with the Romantic philosophers, that: 'the world is so rich that our theories about it will always fail to catch more than a part of it; that there is therefore a range of possible theories about a range of possible processes with regard to epistemologies (and methodologies)'. Law makes a plea for an alternative imagining of methodology that can play with different ways of understanding and representing the multiple, complex realities of the world. Law draws attention to a 'world that is rich in meaning' and that must necessarily resist the attempts to squeeze it into a 'one size fits all' methodology. The task, for Law (2004, p. 6), is to 'respond creatively to a world that is taken to be composed of an excess of generative forces and relations', a world that 'in general defies any attempt at orderly accounting'. Law seeks a method – or more accurately, an idea of 'methodologies' – that allows alternative paths to understandings of social reality.

Central to an understanding of the social foundations of meaning making is the acknowledgement of the relationship between the object of research and the 'knower'. Elizabeth Grosz (1995, p. 28), in writing about the 'crisis of reason', and in her dissection of the presumptions about the criteria by which knowledges are judged valid and/or true, identifies and questions:

> the belief that the object of investigation – whether a text, human behaviour, or social interactions – exists independently of knowledge of it, presuming a reality resistant to false or invalid methods, misinterpretation, or mis-representation … There is, in other words, the presumption of a rift between the object of knowledge and knowing.

The significance of the situated self in the construction of knowledge has been well established, and is accompanied by a firm rejection of the image of the 'view from nowhere' as an idealised conception of objectivity (Nagel 1986). Extending this understanding of the 'knowing subject' Donna Haraway (1991) integrates the embodied self into her concept of situated knowledges, suggesting that as 'knowers' we are always 'located somewhere, in our practices and in our bodies' (cited in Law 2004, p. 68). Law is interested in Haraway's exploration of the significance of the partial connections that emerge, are enacted, at different points of our subjective/social being, and what this means for the construction and enactment of different realities. While recognising the relevance of this to our understanding of how different, necessarily partial, realities are enacted in the various, shifting objects/fields of our research, we are also interested – in much of what follows – in tracing the significance of embodied knowledges for ourselves, as researchers, and for young people, in the construction of meaning in diverse health promotion programs.

Fit to Drive, young people, and embodied health promotion

Over the past few decades schools in many OECD countries, and elsewhere, have become identified as important sites of intervention, targeting young people in relation to health-related issues such as bullying, mental health, eating disorders, same sex attraction, nutrition and physical activity, and sexuality (Colquhoun et al. 1997; Commonwealth Department of Health and Family Services 2000; Crockett 2012; Franze and Paulus 2009; Sheehan et al. 2002; World Health Organisation 2010). Much of this activity reflects the prevalence of ideas about risk, and risk rationalities, that have framed intervention and prevention strategies and programs introduced into schools over the past two decades. Schools have embraced risk frameworks in the formulation of broad policy and program initiatives, and targeted programs and interventions addressing a variety of issues.

As a consequence schools have increasingly become sites for social education, social engagement and the promotion of school welfare, particularly as young people are required to spend longer in secondary education. Schools have become progressively more active in addressing social issues, or observing matters like human rights, though the ways in which they respond to these issues vary significantly (Corney 2006). Moreover, the widening orbit of concerns for schools in relation to duty of care sees them adopting a much more intensive and interventionist role when traumatic events occur, such as road fatalities, in their student population. Fit to Drive sits in this tradition of school-based interventions. As a health promotion program it connects closely with the emerging focus on road safety as a health concern and the positioning of road safety issues and programs in the health promotion field (Montero et al. 2009; Peden et al. 2004). Internationally, schools have been identified in road safety literature as appropriate sites for road safety education (Global Road Safety Partnership 2001).

Schools are generally keen to provide learning opportunities for their students about 'risk' behaviours, specific risks in relation to health and well-being, and road safety and risk. However, the approaches are often dependent on the initiative of individual teachers and the vagaries of the curriculum and extra-curricular pressures. From a school perspective, the Fit to Drive program is unusual in the scope of the exercise – the amount of time and organisation required to stage the event, the degree of staff cooperation and involvement, and the allocation of school space for the day (large group space, break-out rooms). The sheer length of the time devoted to the program – a significant allocation, in the context of school planning – marks it out as an 'event'.

In terms of what it 'does', Fit to Drive is a program based on workshops delivered to year 11 students in a school setting in Victoria, Australia. The workshops tend to look something like this:

A brisk October morning in 2006, in a secondary school on the Mornington Peninsula in Victoria: more than 100 young people are scattered throughout a half dozen seminar rooms adjoining the main school auditorium. A glance into one of these rooms reveals a small group workshop in progress: a group of about 15 to 20 year 11 students are ranged informally around a young facilitator and are vigorously debating the relative riskiness of a set of scenarios displayed on cards on the floor. The students have been invited to rank the scenarios from 'most risky' to 'least risky' and they take turns to rearrange the cards ('driving with a Blood Alcohol Content (BAC) 0.05'; 'speeding in a built-up area', 'driving without a licence'). Sitting in on this activity briefly, I get a sense of the buzz, activity and energetic interaction generated at a Fit to Drive workshop.

Throughout the morning I have noted the contrasts in pace and mood in the half-day program – rowdy exchanges of opinions during a values clarification activity; periods of reflection, and assimilation of new information, during presentations from police; laughter when it looks as if the 'drugs and driving' presenter is going to get them to reveal their own experience with drug use (which doesn't happen, but which grabs the students' attention and involvement from the very start); silently listening to a young woman telling the story of her own loss – her sister had lost her life in a car crash in a spot that would be familiar to the young people present; later in the small groups, working through familiar driving scenarios, working out the risks involved; incorporating their own experience, comparing it with the experience of others, bringing in facts and statistics picked up during the presentations.

I head out onto the practice field with one group of students who are soon jostling for their turn as passengers in the practical safe distance and braking exercise. The students experience first-hand the difference in stopping distances as the driver increases speed on each test run up to 40 kilometres per hour.

Back in the hall gathered in the large group, the final summary aims to give a clear message: 'It doesn't just finish here – stopping the senseless death and injury of our friends and loved ones in road crashes is something we have to take on together and tackle in partnership.' Amid the chaos of students dispersing for lunch break a number of students answer the request for volunteers to be peer leaders. Their task will be to engage with the school community to continue to work on road safety issues in the school, to be the 'eyes and ears' of Fit to Drive, to feed back evidence of raised awareness amongst their peers, and to bring this together at an end of the year forum ('Curbing the Toll').

All of this happens in an environment that emphasises support of, and respect for, the young people and all involved. The presenter who introduces the workshop acknowledges the impact that road trauma has on the whole community and asks participants to take into account the fact that there may be people here who have directly experienced the effects.

Three and a half hours later, the workshop is over for the students, but not yet for the Fit to Drive team. As the students depart the assembly area they receive their showbags and other supporting program material. They hand in evaluation forms and many wave, nod, call out 'thank you', gesturing their appreciation to the team as they leave.

As a morning's program based in a senior secondary school context, Fit to Drive can be functionally written up as a sequence of activities, presentations and small group sessions, with designated time allocations, directions as to where each activity should occur, and who should be conducting each activity. We will introduce and discuss aspects of most, if not all of these activities at different points in what follows. In many respects such an account would mirror or represent any number of other schools based health promotion activities, workshops, interventions. However, this sort of description would not capture the ways in which the whole workshop, in becoming an assemblage of fragments of story, facts, voices, images, movement and personal interactions, becomes in this process an entity that transforms into something that gains its purpose and identity in the particular meshing and correspondence, the flow and flux, of its constituent elements. The combination of stories and other elements cohere momentarily to become something 'other': 'this is precisely what the Deleuzian notion of 'becoming' entails, entry into an arrangement, an assemblage of other fragments, other things, becoming bound up in some other production, forming part of a machine, a component in a series of flows and breaks, of varying speeds and intensities' (Grosz 1995, p. 110).

Although car crashes constitute one of the biggest causes of death and injury for young people, road safety has tended to be overlooked as a concern in adolescent health or health promotion. The area of adolescent health practice and research has tended to focus on biological development, puberty, sexual health, alcohol and other drugs use, mental health, particularly depression and suicide, medical problems common to adolescence (cystic fibrosis, asthma), and treatment and support for young people with chronic illness. In the literature that underpins health policy in Australia, road safety is included in the statistical picture that defines health in terms of mortality, morbidity and, to a lesser extent, 'well-being' (Australian Institute of Health and Welfare 2007, 2011). It has occasionally been mentioned in academic papers as one of the global health challenges in adolescent health (Blum 1988), but practice and program development in the health sector has tended to neglect road safety and continued to principally target more established issues. At a global level road safety is becoming increasingly embedded in the public health agenda. In 2004 the World Health Organisation (WHO) predicted road safety would become the third leading cause of the global burden of disease and injury by 2020, with particular impact in developing countries (Peden et al. 2004; Peden et al. 2008). The United Nations nominated the decade commencing 2011 as the 'Decade of Action for Road Safety' (United Nations 2011). Health promotion conferences have now begun to acknowledge the issue as a global concern (Jong-wook 2006) and health promotion studies cite road safety as an example of the complexity of health issues, and health promotion at the start of the twenty-first century (Balbo 2007).

In the context of other developments in the conceptualisation of health and health promotion over this period, this apparent indifference to road safety issues tends to reveal more about the uneasy political, cultural and bodily space occupied by people's diverse and complex relationships to the car, its association with the so-called 'hard culture' of masculinity (Patience 1992), and the persistence of road trauma's marginalisation as an obdurate problem – 'random events that happen to others' (Peden et al. 2004, p. 2). From the early 1990s concepts of health and young people began to encompass a more holistic approach (in comparison with a single-issue-centred perspective), recognising that issues of self-efficacy, self-care, as well as social environment, play a central role in health outcomes and choices (Rowe et al. 2007; Ioannou et al. 2012). Such factors are also identified as important in relation to road use behaviours and road safety promotion (McQueen and Kickbusch 2007). Recent health promotion discourse has begun to grapple with cultural, as well as social influences impacting on health. Some writers – drawing on Bourdieu's (1990) concepts of 'habitus' – have argued that 'health relevant behaviours are closely linked to broader value systems, behavioural norms, body perceptions' (Abel 2007, p. 43; see also Crawshaw 2004). These, in turn, are produced in environments that maintain unequal distribution of social, economic and cultural resources for the production of health.

Similar issues apply in road safety discourses, and at some points this understanding of road safety as a health promotion issue has connected with the policy goals and strategies of peak health agencies. For instance, the non-government Victorian health promotion organisation VicHealth has recognised road safety as a health issue, supporting programs aiming to develop road safety awareness in specific target groups and communities (RACV/VicHealth 2005). It also developed a partnership with the education unit of the motor vehicle users' member organisation the Royal Automobile Club of Victoria (RACV) that has developed a program based on perceived links between early childhood experience and influences and subsequent driving safety (Vassallo et al. 2007). The RACV/VicHealth Common Solutions project, based on the claim/assumption that 'risky' driving is one characteristic of 'at risk' young people, was initiated in 2005 with the aim to intervene 'upstream' to 'catch' young people who are seen to be at risk of developing clusters of behaviours in childhood and early adolescence which place them at risk of a range of harmful health, education and other life consequences, including road trauma (RACV/VicHealth 2005).

Embodiment and the aesthetics of meaning making

As we have already suggested, John Law (2004, p. 144) argues that social researchers need to let go of certain things in the quest to find new ways of understanding the world – the desire for certainty, the belief in the 'real' as 'relatively stable, determinate, and therefore knowable and predictable'. Young driver discourse as a contested field, a site of vastly differing realities, where the very existence of a 'problem' of young drivers – the very foundation of the Fit to Drive program – may be challenged by different productions of 'realities' that relate to *driving and being young* (see for example Males 2006, 2009). For Fit to Drive the mediation and resolution of this problem – which is a problem of 'knowing' – is critical. To let go of certainty may be sound, and demonstrate a deeper understanding of the nature of 'reality' as 'a set of undecided potentialities … an ultimately undecidable flux' (Law 2004, p. 144). However it must be recognised that we nevertheless face – are required to make – decisions on road safety policy and educational interventions and it is difficult to respond to 'undecidable flux'. Law (2004, p. 144), recognising this paradox, offers a means by which it becomes possible to negotiate this conundrum, by employing the notion of 'method assemblage' to capture, understand and order phenomena. Law's (2004) understanding of method assemblage, rather than overwhelming us with complexity, constant flux and undecidability, allows us a way to explore new understandings, and decide on the 'goods' (such as 'truth', 'politics', 'spirituality', 'justice', 'aesthetics') that might give form, some shape to our analysis, and guide how to act, in a specific time/place/context.

As with all their encounters in/with schooling – via curriculum, pedagogy, knowledge and subject domains, relationships with peers and teachers – the young people in the Fit to Drive workshops bring the outside world to the discursive context of the workshops. Indeed, the workshops are designed around this assumption, building into the educational approach the acknowledgement that young people form their views, values, beliefs and lay the foundations for their behaviours in their diverse, but often shared life-worlds beyond the porous boundaries of school. The 'generative forces' (of their understandings and values) exist in – and beyond – the program. It is difficult, in this sense, to capture and pin down in a static moment a young person's fixed world view, in a setting that is necessarily alive with movement, change, dynamic transaction – 'world-making'. In this context the notion of 'embodied understanding' helps shape the discussion of the aesthetic dimensions of meaning making that we develop in this book: 'Embodying is where being and knowing meet' (Todres 2007, p. 20). Building on philosopher and psychotherapist Eugene Gendlin's (1962, 1995) work to explore the experiential nature of knowing, Les Todres (2007, p. 20) locates the body as being 'interwoven with many realms, the perceptual-textural, the languaged, the affective, the immediately responsive, the interpersonal, the temporal, and even the "unsaid" interweaving of all this together'. Todres writes of the living body that 'inhabits situations intimately' and 'is itself often "lost" out there in the textures, the senses, the flesh, the histories, and the meanings that come from the flowing excess of the lifeworld'. The body also 'carries personal history and prereflective sediments of historical meanings that shape its openness'. However, for Todres (2007, p. 21) a focus on embodied understanding also embraces the idea of partial/relational connections: the lived body is 'full of implicit meanings and relational understanding', and multiplicities. Todres is interested in the body's 'unpacked presences, and its vague, tentative formings', noting that: 'logical language does not like these cracks, whisperings and ambiguities where space/time sequences are not simply sequential'. Todres, takes up the idea that perception is not primary, 'as perception is already based on a distinction between "over there" from "over here" – something important is happening before this spatial distinction in the way that meaning unfolds'. And this 'something important' points to multiplicities and the idea of the 'more': 'the way we are bodily in situations exceeds any precise formulation or patterning of it'.

What Todres (2007, p. 22) calls the 'more' is understood, in part, as an 'interrelated multiplicity'. This is a multiplicity that is 'preseparated', as in prior to separation. This 'more' is 'very fertile', acting as a potential source of 'many strands' of meaning: 'So the body functions in situations as a background knowing of how the situation is as a whole before perceiving its distinctions'. These ideas are of methodological interest here. They provide one means by which we can engage the aesthetic. One means for imagining what might happen if the aesthetic is made present in health promotion with young people, what might happen if the aesthetic is made present in the description, discussion, analysis and critique of health promotion with young people. Both in the implied possibilities for yielding up to the researcher different paths to knowing, as well as in its implications for extending the ideas about how understanding is grounded, not just in language, but in language as 'spoken', enacted in and by the situated, embodied self. We take up these concerns at a number of times in the discussion that follows.

Meaning making here is not about the young people, having previously existed cocoon-like, weaving themselves a personal story about road safety, then 'channelling' it out to be exposed in the workshop, where it is to be neatly challenged or affirmed, or changed. It is rather about the 'production of knowledge' within the Fit to Drive learning environment, and the ways in which the facilitators, the presenters and the other key Fit to Drive actors 'do' diverse things to facilitate the production of that knowledge. In our Prelude we asked the question: *How do we begin to make sense of, and respond to, the loss of young lives on the roads*? This was partly rhetorical. It is also deeply expressive of the mute despair of those affected by road trauma. But the question also speaks to the deeper problem regarding the nature – the possibilities and limits – of knowing. John Law (2004, p. 42) reminds us that there are no certainties, in life, in research, in critique. We must contend with indefiniteness – riding the shifting, unsettled boundaries of 'presence, manifest absence and Otherness' to achieve new ways of knowing. Is there, in the site of young people and road safety, a stable, if not single, narrative that joins the disparate manifestations of 'realities' that will yield 'decidability' – and allow us to act?

Structure of the book

In Chapter 1 we will identify and discuss the ways in which Fit to Drive is aligned with the pedagogical approach of American pragmatist philosopher William James. James appeals to the notion of teaching students to act 'under the notion of a good': a notion that encompasses ideas of responsibility, restraint and care for others. We will argue that it is James' conception of educating for the 'good', as opposed to educating against the 'bad', that most accurately speaks to what the Fit to Drive program is aiming to do in its approach.

A significant part of the workshop intervention aims to move young people away from the notion of 'blame', to the idea of 'responsibility' as a positive 'good'. It promotes the idea that young people are capable (more capable than past generations) of finding solutions to the problem of road trauma. This emphasis on the 'good' is often inevitably overshadowed by the reminders of the 'bad' – grim consequences of crashes, and the negative behaviours associated with crash events. The positive focus on young people's capacity for positive action (good) is asserted in the program's philosophy, expressed in statements such as 'young people have the answers' and 'young people taking responsibility'. It is evident in the efforts to engage young people's 'ownership' through the peer education focus, as well as the organisation of youth forums and initiatives to promote road safety in local communities. Building on this analysis, the chapter will explore what this critique of 'educating for the 'good' may mean for exploring the limits and possibilities of schools based health promotion, and health promotion with young people more broadly.

In Chapter 2 we examine the extent to which the notions and understandings of 'risk', 'risk-taking', and 'at risk' inform and shape the discourse of young people, road use and a whole panoply of concerns with young people's diverse behaviours and dispositions (Kelly 2011). The analysis will contribute to the work that seeks to identify and make problematic the limits and possibilities of imagining young people's health and well-being in terms of risk, of devising and deploying health promotion interventions on the basis of risk discourses and rationalities.

The Fit to Drive workshop incorporates a large group presentation by a police officer, the rationale for which is to 'provide factual evidence about why young people are at risk on the road and how they can be safer road users' (Spencer et al. 2006). This sort of statement signals the key themes of rationality – the adoption of 'safe behaviours' through knowledge of 'facts' – and the mobilisation of risk discourses through which these facts will be interpreted and enacted. In what ways does this framing of health promotion problems connect with contemporary understandings of 'risk'? In what ways does 'risk' inform and shape the way the program gives rational form to, and works with, the prevalence and characteristics of road crashes, and the relationship between young people and the issues associated with heightened crash risk? At many levels the program can be seen as sitting within the tradition of professional interventions that seek to help young risk-takers to 'see the error of their ways and to adopt more "rational" behaviours' (Mitchell et al. 2004, p. 4). Largely absent from this presentation of the 'facts' is any acknowledgement of the pleasures of driving, though the rewards are acknowledged in terms of satisfaction in achievement and new responsibility, one means of marking the passage into adulthood. We will highlight how there is little or no discussion or acknowledgement of the aesthetic appeal of cars, or the sensory pleasures of driving, or the symbolic and cultural significance of the car in contemporary life. The focus is on the car, and driving, as a potential source of danger. The manifest absence, even absence as Other of 'pleasure' from health promotion discourses and interventions has been identified as a limit to promoting behaviour change with young people (Harrison et al. 2011).

In Chapter 3 the focus shifts to two factors that are integral to the ways in which many health promotion interventions attempt to engage with young people's emotional responses to diverse health related issues: through rhetorical strategies such as stories, and through an appeal to 'shared values'. These concerns with emotions and (moral) choices are not peculiar to this program. We will discuss, in a more general sense, how problematising the ways in which emotions and choices are mobilised in health promotion with young people can open up new forms of analysis and critique. This chapter explores the ways that the components of the program – the key messages, emotional engagement and values – are combined in the introductory session to establish the setting for the learning activities. First, Fit to Drive emphasises and engages emotions using oral stories, rhetorical strategies and through short films. Engagement with the emotions is central to young people connecting with the issue and messages, and is, we argue, integral to the reasoning process that the workshop aims to stimulate. The themes of sadness, regret, loss and anger established here are woven throughout the workshop. The second, related, factor is the moral dimension, the engagement with values. The presentation in this section is essentially an attempt to engage the student audience in a sense of shared values around the value of human life, the waste of young lives, and, importantly, questions of personal responsibility and self control. We draw on and use the idea of 'moral emotions' exemplified in the work of Antonio Damasio (1999, 2005), Jack Katz (1999), Mary Midgley (1994, 2003, 2006), Martha Nussbaum (2001a, 2001b) and Mark Johnson (1987, 2007) to discuss how Fit to Drive engages emotions as part of a transformative project.

Chapter 4 explores the facilitated small group session in the Fit to Drive workshop. Facilitated small group discussions are a staple element of much youth work, and much health promotion with young people. We are interested in identifying and exploring the structure, pace and rhythm of small group encounters – the way they 'work'. That is, how the activities are conducted, how they flow, what it is the facilitators do, the place – and the 'work' – of the students. In this chapter we engage with particular phenomenological traditions to explore the relationship between thought/language and bodies/movement, and embodied meaning making in the small group workshop setting. In a contribution to the broader field of health promotion and youth work we will argue that meaning comes into being within the textured experiencing of the 'physical, biological, social, embodied, world' (Johnson 2007, p. 94). Meaning is interactional, and part of the process of experiencing (Gendlin 1962). The interaction occurs not just at the level of the embodied self, but also with/within the social world. Embodied meaning making is inter-relational and inter-subjective, and, in this sense, is always present in health promotion interventions, but often little recognised, little emphasised within the limits of reasoned, rational decision making paradigms. We describe what happens throughout the various workshop activities, and analyse young people's participation in the workshop session, as well as the role and practice of the facilitator, to explore the realm of dialogue, and of language in these types of encounter. We also consider how ideas, thoughts, feelings, reason and rationality are expressed within the physical space of the workshop (emphasising movement, bodies and energy).

In Chapter 3 we argued that the emotional dimension of the workshop is essential to the engagement of young people in the problem of road safety. The fundamental technique of appeal to the emotions is through the medium of story. In Chapter 5 we analyse the role of story-telling within the transformative practices of much health promotion with young people. The role of stories in sense-making, and the generation of meaning, has been explored by many writers (McIntyre 1981; Ochs and Capps 2001; Polkinghorne 1988; Weick 1995). We will draw on this literature, and the insights that emerge from our analysis, to argue that there are profound relations between stories, emotions and choices, that these relations are to be found in much health promotion with young people, and that these relations ought be made explicit in making sense of the limits and possibilities of these types of interventions. The chapter will examine the narrative devices that are a feature of these stories; the impact of 'back-shadowing' and 'fore-shadowing' the events of the story, the place of myth, and the motif of 'journey'. In this chapter we also explore the place of personal narrative, and ask: How do the personal narratives of those who have been affected by road trauma connect with the stories told in Fit to Drive?

Following the police presentation the focus of the workshop is centred on the Metropolitan Fire Brigade's (MFB) presentation of the 'Monavale' case study, based on a crash that occurred in the state of New South Wales, in which two young men were killed. This case study depicts a complex and dramatic story that re/presents a difficult moral tableau that serves to stimulate thinking and debate about responsibility and 'right action' in which each character in the scenario has a moral decision to make, and each workshop participant has to consider that decision in the light of the information that is available to them. From their immersion in the doom-laden story young people must emerge to consider the complexities that are identifiable within this tragedy, and pass judgement on the events and actions of the characters. In Chapter 6 we suggest that the particular power of this and many other stories that are told or emerge from health promotion interventions resonate with the deeply-embedded Western literary traditions of *the tragic*. Central to the dynamic of tragedy, as first established by Aristotle in ancient Greece, and developed in later European traditions of dramatists such as Shakespeare and Schiller, is the interplay of Fate, of individual Character, and the influences of the competing, and complementary, life forces: celebratory, wild Dionysian, and measured, restrained Apollonian. In this chapter we will develop and extend an argument that certain dimensions of young people's health related risks represent, in significant ways, long-standing questions of the struggle between Fate and Reason, the capacity and uses of rationality to impose order from chaos, to assert control in a sea of randomness.

The question of agency, of structure and of the relationships between them is one that continues to trouble youth studies (Kelly 2014). Drawing on literature that critiques the individualisation of risk and the notion of 'choice biographies' Chapter 7 explores the implications – the complexities and dilemmas, as well as the benefits – of positioning young people as 'choosing agents' in relation to road safety, in particular, but also, more generally, in terms of a whole range of concerns with young people's health related behaviours and dispositions. We will explore whether, in the context of the social, economic and cultural realities that limit choice, this is a realistic, or constructive way of thinking about individual (young people's) agency in the context of health promotion, but much more broadly in the context of a globalising, neo-liberal understanding of personhood (Kelly 2013). The chapter discusses and analyses the second facilitated small group session as the workshop takes up the idea of young people as having agency to exercise choice, and to act upon that choice. We analyse the activities, how they work, the dilemmas and difficulties they have presented in practice over the life of the program, and how the young people respond to the activities, particularly in the light of the emphasis on risk logics in the workshop.

This structure makes clear that we have a number of purposes, a number of ends in mind for this description, discussion, analysis, and critique of Fit to Drive, in particular, and school based health promotion in general. But, why is it that we introduce and focus on some things, and not others? Make some things present, some things manifestly absent, still more absent as Other? What are the outcomes, the effects and affects that we have in mind? Our hope is that we will make these ends and purposes clear in what follows. And in our Conclusion we will revisit and consider where, and how, and whether an interest in, and analysis of, the aesthetics of health promotion interventions that target young people allow us to unsettle the limits and possibilities of reason, risk and rationality. At this point, though, John Law (2004), again, provides a means for framing these concerns more broadly than the particular ones that we will identify. As we hinted at earlier, he does this by naming *intent*, or *purpose*, or *concern* as being a *good* (truth, politics, justice, aesthetics ...) that we have in mind to produce through the research, the description, the discussion, the analysis and the critique that we put into play at particular moments. As Law (2004, p. 148) suggests, any methodology, any method assemblage, is *performative* in as much as it *discriminates* 'by trying to enact realities into and out of being'. And in trying to enact different realities in different places and on different occasions, a method assemblage will meet different purposes, produce different effects and different affects: 'This means ... that truth is no longer the only arbiter. No longer, let me stress this, the *only* arbiter'. In describing, discussing, analysing and critiquing Fit to Drive, and school based health promotion with young people, determining the *truth of the matter*, whatever *truth* and *matter* mean in different settings and practices, is something that remains important: '"Is this true?" Yes, this remains a critical question, not one that will go away' (Law 2004, p. 148). As Law (ibid.) further argues:

> method assemblage does not work on the basis of whim or volition. It needs to resonate in and through an extended and materially heterogeneous set of patterned relations if it is to manifest a reality and a presence that relates to that reality. *So truth is a good.*

Law (2004) goes on to argue that in the crafting of method assemblages, the bundling together of the diverse possibilities enabled by the shifting relations between things made present, things made manifestly absent, and things made absent as Other, there is a variety of goods that can be prioritised. Included here are things such as 'politics': 'If politics is about better social ... [and] non-social arrangements, and about the struggles to achieve these, then method assemblage and its products can also be judged politically' (Law 2004, p. 149). There is, always, a politics of presence, manifest absence and absence as Otherness. Law also discusses the ways in which *spirituality* (of a non-religious form), and *justice* are also goods that can inform the crafting of method assemblage. Importantly, for the work we do here, he also highlights the aesthetic dimensions of method assemblage, the possibility that the *aesthetic* is something that, in certain circumstances, for particular purposes, can be included in an ontological politics: 'Thus talk of "beauty" ... or "elegance", or "fit", or "economy" indexes a further set of goods' (Law 2004, p. 149).

While cautioning that 'what counts as beauty can neither be determined in advance, nor out of context', and that 'elegance' and 'beauty' apparently finds a more comfortable place in the talk of physics and mathematics, Law (2004, pp. 149–150) wonders whether the relative absence of a concern with the aesthetic in traditional social science method assemblages 'denies us any grounds for negotiating to enact realities that are true and politically desirable but are also beautiful'. In other words, a disregard for what is understood as the aesthetic 'denies to reality-making any responsibility for beauty, treating this instead as a category error'. As a further caution, one that builds on a sense that *beauty* is itself problematic, our use of the aesthetic will be deliberately ambiguous. A fascist aesthetic, or a Stalinist aesthetic, or a consumerist aesthetic, among many, would, clearly, be suggestive of markedly different things that could be made materially and symbolically present in a vast array of different practices and relations. So our putting into play of the aesthetic will not work to define limits. Rather, we will work to open ways of making meaning that allow certain things to be made present that otherwise might remain manifestly absent, or absent as Other in descriptions, discussions, analyses and critiques of health promotion with young people.

With these possibilities, and limits, in mind we will argue that Fit to Drive, in taking up, reflecting, and remaking the practices and insights of health promotion and moral education, is concerned with not only reducing driving-related risks. It is also aware of the need to build positive values and promote positive environments, including a community of shared values in relation to road safety, which support young people in making safe choices. This involves making meanings that affirm personal safety and care for others, skills to enact safe choices, and an environment that supports this. All of these involve acting for the notion of a 'Good'. The notion of the 'Good' should always be considered problematic. A key means for troubling the 'Good', for imagining what might lie at the limits of reason, rationality and risk in health promotion with young people, is to look to the limits and possibilities that the aesthetic offers for developing and deploying health promotion interventions for young people. This book, we hope, will make a significant contribution to that 'troubling'.

1 School based health promotion as a complex assemblage

In the beginning …

I have made my way down to Madderlake College, on the Mornington Peninsula, for this morning's workshop. Arriving at the school you enter a calm, idyllic environment, with attractive rural surroundings, gently rolling, green hills – a pleasant contrast to the last school I attended which sat uneasily on the dry western plains of Newford, with its flat landscape cut through with eroded gorges, the skyline dominated by planes taking off and arriving at the nearby airport. At Madderlake the still morning is punctuated by the call of magpies and the chirping of New Holland honeyeaters. The school is built into the slopes and contours of the landscape, with moderately-sized buildings nestled into the surrounding grounds, and I keep an eye out for the local kangaroos which I've been assured come here to graze in the early mornings. Stands of eucalypts and mulched beds of native vegetation soften the contours of the paths around the classroom blocks.

The presenters and facilitators arrive early. I meet up with Bern in the car park. She is logistics coordinator for the day, and has already started unloading the facilitators' kits from her car, focussed on the organisational tasks ahead. 'Brooke' has just eased her car into the space beside us and is giving us a cheery wave. An experienced facilitator – she has been working in the program for two years – she will be soon moving into a logistics coordinator role, so will be thinking about the practicalities of organisation as well. Bern strides off, with Brooke and me in tow, to find the workshop venue and the school's Fit to Drive liaison person.

We head to the administration block, where a sign announces 'Reception' through a wide glassed entrance at the end of a timber ramp. This opens on to a bright foyer, with an open plan office behind a counter. The windows and adjacent notice boards are filled with notices, lists, promotional material and posters. A woman behind the glass panels is talking with a female student, whose friend waits nearby. Another reception staff member, seeing us, gets up and opens the other sliding window to help take our enquiry. Hearing our explanation, she directs us to the block where the workshop is being held, across the courtyard, in the auditorium. One of the girls volunteers to take us there, and we are happy to let her lead the way.

We find the Madderlake coordinator, Jillian, who is the school welfare officer, greeting people and arranging coffee. Graham is there with an observer from another road safety organisation and he is anxious for me to meet her – politics are never far from the agenda. The absence of some students, who are unexpectedly on an excursion, is disappointing for Jillian. This is her last year as coordinator and she is anxious for the day to be a success. The atmosphere is generally relaxed, however. Jill has organised morning tea for the whole year group, people are happy to see each other, and they take time to greet each other, shake hands and give each other a hug.

The introductory session for this workshop takes place in the semi-formal setting of the comfortably-sized multi-purpose school auditorium. It will be the venue for the whole-group activities of the workshop – the introduction, presentations and final wrap-up. The auditorium is used for dramatic and musical productions, as well as the formal business of school life, and boasts the miscellaneous trappings of the theatre – lights, cables, scenery stacked against one wall – along with lectern, table, portable screen and speakers' chairs.

The facilitators are chatting in their own group across the room. There are six here today, five young women, and Brad, who has been recently trained. It's always good to have young males in the group. Nearly all of the facilitators are tertiary students, with Gracie, who works part-time in local government youth services, the only non-student. The facilitators are dressed in the favoured style – jeans or pants, sweaters, tops and cardigans. They look comfortable, inconspicuous and achieve just the right note of informality. This impression is reinforced by their quiet presence in the auditorium. The other visitors, however, provide an interesting contrast. A mix of suits and blue uniforms. The blue uniforms belong to Barry, and the MFB officers. Dressed with slightly less formality are the local government's road safety officer and roadsafe committee representatives, who are there to run an activity demonstrating car braking and stopping distances. Bern has time for a quick greeting before getting straight into organising mode. As logistics coordinator for the workshop she needs to immediately check in with the facilitators, and consult with them about the specific arrangements for the morning. She needs to ascertain how many year 11 students there will be (around 100), how they'll be divided into groups, where the rooms are, and allocate the facilitators to the groups. She needs to work out the sequencing of workshop activities – there is always slight variation to allow for two groups at a time to go out to do the car braking exercise. I leave her some space to speak with the facilitators, and they're soon huddled around her. The image it brings to mind is of a football coach at half-time, clip-board in hand, gesticulating (I think she's pointing out the open space where the car braking exercise will be), pointing out something in her notes (the workshop schedule perhaps, adjusting the times to accommodate the car braking activity). The facilitators listen intently, with an occasional question or comment.

Before long there is a sense that things are about to start, people are winding up their conversations and looking around for signs that they should be moving into place. The facilitators take seats along the front row, and I join them, a little to the side so I can see the students as well as the presentation. Altogether, counting the MFB, VicPolice, Graham, Jillian the school liaison person, Bern as logistics coordinator, the six facilitators, the visitor from the Road Trauma group and me, there are fifteen people milling around the front of the hall. For the young people, some of whom are now starting to gather outside the door – we see some peering through, making faces and jostling around – there are fourteen completely new faces to take in. More students have started to arrive, coming from their home groups, where they spend the first ten minutes of the day. A couple stand at the doorway, peering through. One asks if they're allowed to come in now. The dribble of students turns into a stream, and the hall fills with the hubbub of chatter, laughter, a bit of pushing and shoving, with remonstrations from the teachers accompanying them. There are about four teachers with them, who encourage, direct and shepherd the students to take their seats. The demeanour of the students is mixed – chatty, boisterous, excited, nonchalant, some dragging their feet, occupied with their own concerns. At the same time they are checking out the new (Fit to Drive) people, mostly demonstrating friendly curiosity.

The students, I note irrelevantly, are colour-coordinated with the MFB and police: a sea of dark blue uniforms. Among the students' uniformity, there's a note of informality, individual touches, an artful deconstructing of the uniform. Some girls wear their skirts über-long, shin-length. Students muffled in colourful scarves, blowing on chilled fingers through fingerless gloves, hair streaked with blue or red, as well as the ubiquitous blonde streaks (for both boys and girls), boys' shirts hanging out, ear-rings dangling through their ears, various ingenious arrangements of socks.

The students are seated by this time and are looking down on the presenters from the tiered seating, which a speaker could find intimidating, I'd imagine. The formality of the setting, however, is tempered by the casual atmosphere that is created by the relaxed and friendly interaction among the Fit to Drive presenters and facilitators, and the Fit to Drive personnel and school staff.

Once the students are seated and settled Jillian introduces the workshop presenters and facilitators, and gives a brief background to the school's involvement with the program. 'This,' she explains, 'is the eighth year the school has been running the Fit to Drive program. We were one of the first schools to run the workshop, so have had a long commitment to the program and the effort to keep young people safe on the roads.' She points out the number of people who have come to the school today committed to this very purpose, and asks the students to make the team welcome. She then hands over to Graham, who will be doing the introduction today.

Graham manages to convey both energy and relaxed ease as he takes the floor. Introducing himself, pausing dramatically for effect – 'Graham Spencer's the name … I'm a former school principal – and don't I look it!' – his friendly smile seems to belie the implications of the image he conjures – THE school principal. Authoritative, if not authoritarian; embodying status and authority, no nonsense. This image is reinforced by his physical appearance: neatly dressed, in a conservative, well-cut grey suit, immaculately presented. Tie precisely knotted and in place, shoes polished, every hair on his greying, well-barbered head in place. The suit, he jokingly acknowledges, is part of his persona – his students used to say they 'wouldn't be able to recognise him without his tie'. He gives a sketch of his background, mentioning the neighbouring school where he was a principal for nearly ten years. Some students nod in recognition of the school. Some smile and nudge their neighbours.

And so the school based intervention begins…

In this chapter we want to develop and explore a framework for situating Fit to Drive, and other school based health promotion interventions, as being structured, in diverse ways, by often complex and competing ideas about 'the Good' (James 2010). Embedded in the logic of these programs, in ways that are manifested differently, is a sense that the intervention wants to, promises to, produce better health and well-being outcomes for young people, and, often, for their families, their communities, even the 'nation'. These 'goods' are not unproblematic in so far as both the ends, the 'goods', and the means for producing these ends, are often, usually, subject to significant discussion and debate. But a particular view of the 'good' that invests meaning and purpose in a particular program can be made apparent, can be analysed and interpreted, can be critiqued. Part of what we will argue here is that the 'good' that might shape and be produced in a particular school based health promotion intervention is necessarily limited by its location in a school, in the institutionalised and regulated spaces of schooling. The school, any and all schools, can be understood, following Foucault, as a necessarily limited field of possibilities in which some things are thinkable, or do-able, or possible. And others not.

Drawing on and further developing John Law's (2004) idea of a method assemblage, we will explore the ways in which school based health promotion is a particular, though complex assemblage in which an array of spatial relations and spaces, actors and agencies, knowledges, practices and power relations make some things possible, others not possible. Makes some things present, other things manifestly absent, still more things absent as Other. Much of the work we will do in thinking about health promotion as a complex assemblage will unfold in later chapters, in later discussions of risk, of values, of stories, of Greek tragedy. In this chapter we begin this work by setting the scene for a school based intervention by 'rethinking the school' in ways that draw on the work of Ian Hunter and Nikolas Rose. Rethinking that also draws on work we have done elsewhere (for example, Pike and Kelly 2014). Here we also engage with the ways in which William James discusses 'educating for the good', and the ways in which John Law argues that research and analysis and critique (the work we do here) might produce a variety of 'goods', including but not limited to, 'truth', 'politics', 'justice', 'aesthetics'.

The 'irreal' spaces of schools

The half-day workshop is an event clearly requiring high levels of organisation. In some regions, the spectacle is reinforced through activities outdoors, such as practical demonstrations of car braking and stopping distances. A large team of people is assembled here, and the impact of the group coming together at the beginning of the workshop – the facilitators, logistics coordinator, presenter/s, plus school personnel – is impressive. The students have the sort of reactions observed in any audience: curiosity, interest, anticipation, bored nonchalance.

Schools as institutions are generally familiar and unchanging. On a day-to-day basis schools present few surprises or novelties for students and staff. Whether government or non-government run, wealthy or struggling, schools tend to share certain features. Large bodies of students organised into year groupings and assigned to designated physical spaces; routines established by class schedules, often marked by ringing of bells. Most schools in Victoria (Australia) have a school uniform policy, more or less strictly enforced. And students, more or less rebelliously, deconstruct those uniforms, with alterations and embellishments. Any new event or sight provides a distraction and interrupts the routine. Schools periodically involve outsiders in the classroom or programs, to bring specialist knowledge and links for the young people to resources outside the school, and in recent years there has been an increased focus on increasing the community–school interface, but usually these initiatives don't make much of a dent in the school routine (DEECD 2007).

The first sight of the Fit to Drive visitors is thus a combination of the familiar and the novel. The familiar is signalled by the school setting, the teachers, the notion of occasional visitors bringing knowledge deemed to be useful to students. At the same time, the first sight of unfamiliar visitors in the school arouses curiosity and friendly interest in students. The appearance of police and other official vehicles in the car park adds to a sense of drama.

For the year 11 students, there has been some preparation in anticipation of the Fit to Drive program. They have been informed of the change in timetable, and that the whole morning will be set aside for a road safety program. They have also been allocated into special groups ahead of time. In the schools where they will be involved in a car braking activity, the young people have been required to return permission forms. For some of the teachers, there will be some annoyance that this workshop will be taking time away from their normal class time. The extensive/intensive demands on a crowded curriculum are increasingly an issue for schools and teachers, but many will welcome the road safety education for their students. Many will take it as some welcome time out from the classroom, and a chance to catch up on marking and preparation.

The fact that two thirds of the year 11 school day is allocated to the workshop is in itself significant and unusual. Unlike other programs that are designed to be taught by the classroom teacher within specific subject areas,

Fit to Drive is a 'whole school curriculum approach' (Rowe et al. 2007; Montero and Spencer 2009). As such it is not syphoned off into the curriculum of an isolated subject area. It sits outside the usual topic/subject 'silos'. Involving the students as a whole year group, the program requires, and is designed around, the commitment of the school leadership to its implementation, although it may rely on a 'champion' within the school itself. This role of 'champion' may be taken up by staff in varied roles, from year-level coordinators to deputy principal, to an engaged and committed individual classroom teacher. The effort involved in this project of 'championing' the program in individual schools is alleviated by the existence and support of the broader Fit to Drive community.

Here we deliberately use 'community' rather than 'organisation'. Usually the contact with the program will be through the Fit to Drive Local Area Coordinator (LAC), who will probably have a long history of connection with both the local community and schools in the area. This may be in their role of school–community liaison, their background as key school figure, or their involvement in local government or community organisations. Often the school 'champion' will have had a direct involvement in local road safety initiatives, such as the community road safety committee, and they will know the local police Youth Resource Officers (YROs), or fire officers, or even some of the facilitators who will be delivering the program in their school. This local network is in turn connected with the broader 'community of interest' of road safety. It is through this web of local relationships and sense of place that the tightly scripted and managed program transforms into a 'living', organic entity.

Elsewhere we (Pike and Kelly 2014) have discussed the ways in which the problem of school based meals provision to children and young people in places such as the UK, the USA and Australia can be understood in terms of the spaces and behaviours, the policies and practices, the 'lines of force' that construct and traverse the 'moral geographies of children, young people and food'. Put simply, the dining rooms of UK, US and Australian schools (and elsewhere) can be conceived as 'battlegrounds' in which a wide array of actors, agencies, knowledges, histories and spaces make, enact and transform understandings of the different rights, responsibilities and obligations of young people and families, teachers and schools, the state, and large, often multinational, food companies in relation to food, diet and young people's health and well-being. In these spaces the moral project of government seeks to render knowable the problems of young people, food practices, diet, health and well-being in ways that make different actors and agencies and organisations differently responsible for different aspects of this problem. And, in spaces such as schools, this problem can only be made knowable within particular limits and possibilities. Two concepts that we introduced in that discussion are useful to the work that we want to do in this chapter: the idea that schools need to be made as 'governable spaces', and the idea that the subjects of government need to be made knowable in ways that promise to make them governable.[1]

Our discussion there made reference to Michel Foucault's (1991) later work on government to focus on the productive dimensions of schooling, of relations, of government, of space. We considered the ways in which the different governmental aspirations related to health, education, welfare and the production of healthy, self-governing young people are brought together in the school dining room – to shape that space, and, in turn, to be shaped by that space. We drew on Ian Hunter's (1994) genealogy of mass compulsory schooling, and Nikolas Rose's (1999) *Powers of Freedom*, to conceptualise schools as governable spaces that have been made 'real' for an array of purposes, and in less than ideal circumstances.

Understood in this way we can think about the ways in which schools, and school spaces such as dining rooms, are mobilised in always contingent, more or less successful attempts to meet particular ends such as the development of young people who are capable of making healthy choices about food. This framework, as we will see, enables us to make a similar argument in relation to the 'staging', the spaces, the relations and practices, the players involved in Fit to Drive's attempts to provoke in young people the capacity to make better choices in relation to driving and road safety practices.

Ian Hunter's (1994) *Rethinking the School* draws on aspects of Foucault's concepts of government in a 'genealogical' contribution to debates about what schools should do, what their purposes are, and the reasons why they might not achieve these *ideals*. Hunter is also interested in examining the *positions* from which these debates are carried out. His examination highlights the *principled positions* adopted by some of the critics of mass, compulsory, state regulated schooling and its apparent failure to meet the higher purposes outlined by these critics. Hunter argues that many of these critics (radical, conservative, feminist, religious) fail to take account of the history of mass compulsory, state regulated schooling. A history that is marked by things such as the following: a lack of unity of purposes for schooling; the limited ways that are available for thinking about education (political rationalities); the limited techniques that are available for educating large numbers of children and young people (governmental technologies). As Hunter suggests, schools have never existed in their *ideal* form, and as we live in a *less than ideal* world they probably never will. It also means that we will, and should, continue to have arguments about schools and their purposes – but on what terms? Hunter's genealogy is instructive in making clear the contingent, limited and often shared understandings of what might be called the moral project of schooling that drove early, nineteenth-century attempts in the UK to develop a compulsory, state regulated system for the education of the children of the masses. For example, here he is citing an early nineteenth-century factory inspector who is clear about the 'moral project' that schooling should serve:

> To put the necessity of properly educating the children of the working classes on its lowest footing, it is loudly called for as a matter of policy, to

> prevent a multitude of immoral and vicious beings, the offspring of ignorance, from growing up around us, to be a pest and a nuisance to society; it is necessary in order to render the great body of the working class governable by reason.
>
> (Hunter 1994, p. xi)

He further cites William Lovett's 'radical' hope for a 'school system that was democratically organised and dedicated to human emancipation'. A radical vision, a 'good', that must not, nevertheless, be left to chance:

> While much moral instruction may be conveyed in the school-room, the playground will be found the best place for moral training, where all [the children's] faculties will be active, and when their dispositions and feelings will all be displayed in a different manner than when they are in the school-room, where silence, order and discipline should prevail. But when in the playground, the teacher should incite them to amusement and activity, in order to develop their characters.
>
> (Hunter 1994, xi–xii)

And, in startlingly similar tones, a middle class reformer's view of what the space of a well governed and regulated playground offered to those interested in the education and moral training of the *poorer* classes:

> A playground is in fact the principal scene of the real life of children … the arena on which their true character and dispositions are exhibited; and where, free and unrestrained, they can hop and jump about, swing, or play at tig, ball, or marbles …
>
> Amidst this busy scene, the trainer must be present, not to check but to encourage youthful gaiety. All is free as air, and subject only to a moral observation of any particular delinquency, the review of which is reserved for the school gallery, and taken up on the children's return there, and pictured out as a moral training lesson.
>
> (James Kay Shuttleworth, submission to Select Committee on the Education of the Poorer Classes, cited in Hunter 1994, xiii)

As we suggested in our discussion of the moral geographies of children, young people and food (Pike and Kelly 2014), government is not just the about imposition of your will in 'the real'. The William Lovetts, James Kay Shuttleworths, the factory inspectors, the critics of schooling, all may have ideas and ideals in relation to schooling and the 'making up' of self governing, autonomous, choice making children and young people. In this sense, government is productive. However, government is also technical. It depends on being able to think and act in ways that promise to make government possible. Government, in this sense, is fundamentally about 'timetables', 'committees', 'structures', 'rules', 'resources' …

This sense of the arts of government as being, to a significant degree, a technical enterprise, a series of practices in which the means for producing ends/goods are always limited; always, to some extent, contextual; always subject to economic considerations; also, inevitably, extends to the 'subjects' of government. To those children and young people who need to be guided, directed, encouraged, cajoled to develop, and put into play, a variety of behaviours and dispositions – in relation to diet and food practice, road safety, sexualities, alcohol and drug use. As Nikolas Rose (1999) demonstrates, modern practices of government are dependent on making the subjects of government *knowable*. For governmental programs to deliver their 'goods' we need to know who is to be governed, and we need to construct an understanding of their behaviours, attitudes, desires, habits and hopes – all in relation to the problem of government that is being addressed by a particular strategy:

> Are we to be governed as members of a flock to be led, as children to be coddled and educated, as a human resource to be exploited, as members of a population to be managed, as legal subjects with rights, as responsible citizens of an interdependent society?
>
> (Rose 1999, p. 41)

Governmentality studies have demonstrated that the 'ideal' subject of liberal government is the self reflecting, self fashioning individual who has developed the capacity to control the *impulsive, passionate* and *desiring* aspects of human behaviour (Kelly 2013; Pike and Kelly 2014). This capacity is something that is not seen to be innate. It is a capacity, or human behaviour, that has to be encouraged, incited and produced through education and moral training. In liberal and neo-liberal mentalities of rule the capacity for self control has been, and is, used to 'differentiate – the child from the adult, the man from the women, the normal person from the lunatic, the civilized man from the primitive' (Rose 1999, p. 44). It is in this sense that we (Pike and Kelly 2014) cited Rose's (1999, p. 45) suggestion that the historical development of mass compulsory schooling, and the practices and processes that give it structure, that give form to a school day – 'from breaks for recreation in the playground supervised by the teacher as moral exemplar, to the introduction of literary education to inculcate the habits of self-reflection and inwardness' – can be understood as 'technologies of moral training'. The promise of such technologies was that 'the child acquired the habits of self-observation and self-regulation in everyday existence outside the classroom'.

In addtion, we suggested that government does not take place in some 'pre-existing thought world' with its own 'natural divisions' (Rose 1999, p. 32). As Rose (ibid.) argues, government is an activity that requires human experience to be subdivided, so to speak, by time and space. Government occurs across different 'time zones'. In schools these 'zones' include the school day, week, term, year, and out-of-school hours. And in different 'spaces of government' such as the classroom, the staff room, the head teacher's office, the canteen, the school yard, the playground, the school dining room. These 'time zones' and 'spaces of government' are not natural phenomena. They have to be thought about (rationalised) and brought into being, made real, as times and spaces appropriate to particular tasks of government. In this way, schools – with their timetables that break the day up into governable bits and the curriculum that divides knowledge up into knowable bits – have been built as governable spaces in which the making up of desirable behaviours and attitudes in young people might be readily accomplished.

It is in this sense also that Rose (ibid.) suggests that these fabricated spaces, these governable spaces are 'irreal': 'there is no independent access to one true world against which our versions of it can be compared … All we have are different versions of the world … constructed out of words, numerals, pictures, sounds or symbols'. This irreality should not be seen to be somehow less 'real' than the 'real world'. In this way of imagining the school as an assemblage of time zones and governable spaces there is no place for that mythical 'real world' often invoked in spaces such as schools and universities ('In the real world …'; 'Learning for the real world …'). Rather, different spaces are made real in diverse ways, and in various forms of relationships with other spaces whose own reality is given a particular shape, a particular character that is more or less fit for particular purposes. Rose's (1999, pp. 32–33) own irrealism is technical. Government becomes possible, he argues, 'only through discursive mechanisms … This is a matter of defining boundaries, rendering that within visible, assembling information about that which is included and devising techniques to mobilize the forces and entities thus revealed'.

In this way we suggested that thinking about 'the moral geographies of young people and food' meant that we should approach the school, and understand it, as an assemblage consisting of, among other things: time zones and governable spaces; a less than ideal history, present and future; an array of actants (human and non-human) with complementary but often competing interests; a historically informed, sometimes shifting, but always limited range of ways to imagine the purposes of schooling; and a contingent and limited set of technologies with which to make things happen, to meet these purposes.

In a similar vein to the work we did there, we want to spend some time now locating Fit to Drive in the 'time zones' and 'irreal spaces' of different schools. In doing this work we open up Fit to Drive to a form of analysis in which those things that are present, that are manifestly absent, are absent as Other, might be made apparent.

'Take any empty space …': transforming the space, becoming theatre

The settings for Fit to Drive workshops are many and diverse. Whether auditorium or library foyer, traditional gloomy school hall, or bright, modern multi-purpose space, a common feature of the workshop is the theatricality of the opening session.[2] The sessions are resided over by the 'master of ceremonies' [sic], a role with resonances of ritual, the observance of ceremony and dramatic forms. The master of ceremonies – in the example we use it is Graham – is a familiar character, translated into a slightly unfamiliar context. His appearance, presence, and even his joking references, identify him as a principal 'type'. In this sense he is a stock character on the school 'stage'. In other respects his appearance presages a special event. The presence of someone of the status of principal indicates that the action to follow is accorded some importance.

Peter Brook (1996, p. 5) powerfully captures the fundamental conditions for an event to be experienced as theatre: 'I can take any empty space and call it a bare stage. A man walks across this empty space while someone else is watching him; and this is all that is needed for an act of theatre to be engaged'. This, for Brook, is the starting point for an act of theatre. In the schools the space that is the setting for the large group session of the workshop is transformed on each occasion into a space for the staging of the Fit to Drive performance – an 'intentional re-allocation and semiotization of space' (Montelle 2009, p. 5). The stage, or auditorium, or multi-purpose room, is transformed into an 'intentional space', and the presenter inhabits that space in a manner that signals the commencement of a ceremony, and performance. The transformed space, and the person in that space, commands a particular attention from the audience. The attention – the energy, as Brook (1996) would describe it – of the audience is drawn towards that person.

In his *The Presentation of Self in Everyday Life*, Erving Goffman (1980) drew on dramaturgical metaphors to explore the idea of the self as a managed performance undertaken by individuals in the context of everyday social interaction. Goffman's analysis suggests an initial starting point for reflecting on the nature of the relationship between the presenter/master of ceremonies and the audience of year 11 students (and teachers) in Fit to Drive. Graham's arrangement of his performance in the context of the opening 'scene' involves a pronounced awareness of, and deliberate playing to, the image he projects, and the anticipated 'audience' response to this. Graham enters into a reflexive relationship with the audience that is characterised on the one hand by his attention to the management of the performance to achieve certain ends, and on the other by acceptance, on the part of the audience, of the 'part' he is performing in this situation (Goffman 1980, p. 28). However we interpret this scene, the drama of the moment is palpable, a reminder of the power of drama as 'a medium of mass communication that can be adapted to almost any message or purpose' (Csapo 2010, p. xi).

Goffman (1980, p. 246) reflexively adopted the language of the stage as his conceptual framework to interpret the 'structure of social encounters', with the acknowledgement that the theatrical analogy was an interpretive and rhetorical device, and that he was not concerned with 'aspects of theatre that creep into everyday life'. Montelle (2009, p. 5), who explores the 'ubiquity of theatricality' as a prelude to his study of the emergence of theatricality as social practice, distinguishes between fundamentally divergent ideas of theatricality emanating from different academic traditions. He takes issue with what he terms the 'trivialisation' of the idea of theatricality as defined by certain sociological traditions represented, or influenced, by Goffman. This trivialisation is achieved, according to Montelle (2009, p. 20) 'by turning the word into a generic term describing any performative action in the complex world of everyday life'. This, he maintains, neglects the essential character of theatricality, and the defined role of theatre as a purposefully constructed semiotic space, involving intentional spatial and iconographical practices (Montelle 2009, p. 5). In the Fit to Drive workshop, immediately the presenter 'takes the stage', it is evident that we are seeing a performance within the recognisable iconography of theatrical convention. The presenter projects voice, and bodily presence. Gestures and movement are controlled, almost stylised at times. They are 'theatrical' gestures. Later, during the telling of a story that had significant personal impact, these symbolic gestures will allow the presenter to powerfully convey, without 'succumbing' to emotion. In a sense, the adopted (and recognisable) repertoire of gestures shields the performer from fully re-experiencing that emotion and thus losing control – and authority – as presenter/performer.

Understandings of theatre as institution (Montelle 2009), and theatricality and performance as social practice (Goffman 1980), inform our interpretation of the introductory session of Fit to Drive as theatre. Theories accounting for the origins of theatre, though contested (Csapo and Miller 2007; Rozik 2002), are relevant here. Eli Rozik (2002), for example, identifies theatre as a medium, as a specific form of human communication and creative expression, as emanating from the fundamental condition of the human psyche, indeed, the very structure of the human brain and its capacity to think in images and symbols. This is theatre interpreted as an expression of human creative thought and aesthetic sensibilities, but more fundamentally of an innate human faculty of thinking as a form of creative imagining: 'theatre is a specific imagistic medium (i.e., a method, or, rather, an instrument of thinking and communication), and as such its roots lie in the spontaneous image-making faculty of the human psyche' (Rozik 2002, p. xi). For Rozik (2002, p. 47) the roots of theatre emerge from 'the human brain's inbuilt capacity to create images and think by means of them'. Theories of symbolic and imagistic thinking inform this view. Rozik discusses Susanne Langer's contribution to theories of symbolic and imagistic thinking and their relevance for theories of theatre origins. For Langer, images are 'our readiest instruments for abstracting concepts from the tumbling stream of actual impressions. They make our primitive abstractions for us, they are our spontaneous embodiments of general ideas' (Langer, cited in Rozik 2002, p. 247). Central to this idea of theatre is the suggestion that thinking is essentially symbolic in form – a characteristic that lends itself to forms of theatrical expression.

Dismissing theories that identify theatre's origins in ritual – 'theatre is a medium, ritual is a mode of action' – Rozik (2002, p. x) argues that ritual, 'as a complex of cultural activities, can not only display elements of theatre, but also draw upon other arts, such as storytelling, music, dance, design, sculpture and architecture'. Theatre and ritual are 'entities on different levels of human activity' which 'operate on different ontological levels' (Rozik 2002, p. 337).

While the nuanced arguments surrounding the question of theatre's origins in ritual may remain unresolved, and are perhaps unresolvable, in theatre studies, the evidence for deep associations between ritual and theatre illuminate some of the features of both that appear in Fit to Drive. Ritual, according to Rozik (2002, p. 337), may be understood as 'a complex text that combines several methods of signification and communication, including body language and verbal and iconic media, in literal and metaphorical capacities'. Such a complex text is 'aimed at achieving special effects in the divine or other sphere for the benefit of a real community'. For Rozik (2002, p. 338), it is *acting* that is the distinctive characteristic of theatre:

> Acting is always characterized by a fundamental duality, of which the audience is always aware: actors performing a text, which they inscribe on their own bodies, and descriptions of real or fictional characters distinct from themselves. Even actors acting themselves are distinct from their real selves and from anyone projecting an image of themselves in real behaviour.

In this sense Graham is both an 'actor acting himself' and at the same time playing a 'part' in the context of a complex social interaction, and managing complex 'dramaturgical discipline' in his 'presentation of self' (Goffman 1980).

Whatever the explanations of its origins, throughout human history theatre, in its various forms, has become a protected ('sacred') and stylised space for the expression, and working through, of human existential struggles, of social and cultural tensions, the airing of devils, the transmission of values and reinforcement of taboos. The development of theatrical forms for the exploration of matters of human significance has grown out of, and continues to be connected with, socio-cultural and socio-economic conditions. One of the eternal themes of theatre is the exploration of the relationship of individual to community – a central concern of Fit to Drive. The theatrical element of the Fit to Drive introductory session recalls that theatre may serve a function in the forging of community, around shared stories within a ritual space. The space for this shared exploration is firmly established in the coming-together of audience and presenter/performer in the opening session of the program. The 'community' that is forged in a Fit to Drive workshop is a reflection/refraction of the broader community to which performers, participants and audience belong – a community that, they will learn, can be fractured in multiple ways through the impacts of often fatal road trauma.

One of the fundamental conditions for an act of theatre to exist is the presence of an audience (Fischer-Lichte 2005; Hartnoll 2003; Montelle 2009). The audience/observer is the 'decoder of intention' (Montelle 2009, p. 5). The relationship between audience and performance, and performance space, is dynamic, and productive of meaning. The transformation of individual – and straggling groups of – year 11 students into an 'audience' is achieved through a gathering (Law 2004) of such things as the following: the students entering into the defined, ceremonial, space of the event; the setting, the intentions of the presenters, signalled by preparations on stage; and the energy generated within the bodily co-presence of performer and audience/spectator in the space (Fischer-Lichte 2005). This effect is reinforced when presenters move into the audience to engage with some of the students beforehand, thereby establishing connection, perhaps gleaning information they can use to connect with the audience in their opening. In this way the ground is prepared for the students/audience to play their role in the event, as the presenter/narrator conveys their message, through stories, and later when they engage more actively in the small group sessions. When the drama and conflict is played out on the screen, in the filmed stories and interviews, this is grounded in the presenter's narration, and the bodily co-presence of audience, facilitators, teachers and other presenters. It is also shaped by the materiality of the space.

The players in a school based performance

The other significant feature immediately apparent to the students and school staff is the number and variety of personnel involved in delivering the program. Involved in the event at Madderlake College are officers from Victoria Police (youth resource officers), the Metropolitan Fire Brigade (MFB), a local government road safety department, and VicRoad's local Road Safety Committee. On other occasions there may be a guest speaker from the Teenage Road Accident Group – a community group of those affected by road trauma – or other volunteer speakers. Behind the scenes support for the program has come from organisations involved in road safety education, such as the RACV,[3] the Transport Accident Commission (TAC), the Department of Education and Early Childhood Development (DEECD), Country Fire Authority (CFA), and the government roads authority, VicRoads.

In Victoria over the past decade or so there have been numerous school based road safety programs developed that target different school population groups, from primary to secondary, junior and senior years (see for example VicRoads 2006). These, no less than other health promotion initiatives, have characteristically been dependent on staff resources, interest and expertise, and space within the crowded school curriculum, with the result that road safety may have been implemented in an *ad hoc* and inconsistent fashion. The Fit to Drive program has been able to provide a platform for the coordination of these resources and programs. Rather than competing for contested space in the curriculum, the coordinated approach, as well as the growing influence of Fit to Drive, led to a more consistent presence of these road safety organisations in schools. The major stakeholders of the Victorian Government's

'Arrive Alive' strategy (Arrive Alive 2012), namely VicPolice, VicRoads, the TAC, DEECD, RACV, the MFB and CFA, local councils and community road safety education groups, increased their presence in secondary schools by means of their participation in the program. Resource considerations are always present. Although competition for finite road safety education resources is part of the reality of organisational operation, the practical 'pooling' of organisational resources around the Fit to Drive workshop adds to the sense of community.

By the time the students and staff have started making their way to the auditorium, the curiosity is starting to register. What do the students see?

As they settle in they are presented with a whole new sea of faces, a novelty that immediately attracts their interest and anticipation. Among the suits and the uniforms there is the more youthful appearance of the facilitators, not much older than themselves. Facilitators in training have been reminded that, from the moment they arrive in their car, they are role models; they are being observed: 'The young people are watching you', they are told in training. The employment of 'trained tertiary students as role models' and workshop facilitators is promoted as a distinctive feature of Fit to Drive (Spencer and Montero 2011). Facilitators (and presenters) have to 'present' an image – responsible, caring for others, enthusiastic – and *be* that image throughout the morning. This includes, of course, driving carefully and demonstrating respect for the school and community environment.

Facilitators are asked to dress 'neat and casual'. Bare midriffs, ripped jeans – of the non-designer type – belly rings and the like (which did turn up occasionally in the beginning) are, they are gently reminded, distracting and present an unprofessional image. The focus is on the students: 'It's not about you, it's about the students.' At the same time their style makes a statement about the program's intentions and their role in it. Facilitators are not strictly 'peer' in age, maturity, and life experience and circumstances. The promise is that barriers of age and style, and power relations, are shifted, at least a little. The facilitators immediately stand out as different to school staff and the usual visitors, a fact that students often remark on in their feedback.

So, as the students wait they may be looking at the dynamic interplay between the people on the stage – relaxed conversation, or more intense discussions; small dramas focussed on the equipment, checking of watches. Or they may be focussing on the group of facilitators sitting in the front as they conduct their own whispered conversation, or wait quietly, checking notes. Soon, something seems to be happening; the school coordinator is calling for hush, and makes ready to introduce the visitors, and the presenter.

Earlier in this chapter we described Graham's first interaction with the students, the use of mildly self-mocking humour to stimulate connection and interest and to focus attention. This is an important moment in the task of engaging the audience, a preparation for the serious message and shift in tone that is now to come with his story to follow. In a later chapter we analyse the role of stories in Fit to Drive, arguing that stories are the key technique of engagement, meaning making and creation of shared values in relation to the problem of road trauma in the program. A story, no matter how powerful and affecting in itself, does, in the end, need to be told. Part of the 'tellership' (Bakhtin 1981) of a story is the status of the 'teller'. Are they credible? Do they convey authority? Do they have 'presence'? In Fit to Drive the introductory stories have typically been told by someone who is manifestly an authority figure, in a space that has associations with theatre and ritual. In the telling of the Fit to Drive stories there are inevitable questions of performance involved, especially in the presentation of the large group information sessions. The impact of the story is dependent on the effectiveness of the presenter as performer. Even as the focus is on engaging the participation of the students, 'handing over' to the students and politically downplaying the role of the presenter, the presenter has a pivotal role.

'*Close your eyes. I want you imagine this …*' Alison the CFA presenter instructs the gathered students, as she prepares to set the scene for the Monavale crash re-enactment at one of the workshops.[4] The students obediently close their eyes, or bow their heads. Not many refuse to comply, and those who do find themselves surrounded by fellow students who aren't paying attention to them. In this way Alison is able to quickly lead the students into an imagined world where they will be focussed on the story of the young people at Monavale.

Other presenters use the space in creative ways to tell the story. They might involve 'audience participation' by bringing students up to take part in aspects of the presentation. They might move into the group, shifting the focus of attention. Jarrad from the MFB, when telling the story about the Monavale crash, sets the scene with the use of props, arranging chairs to re-create the 'car', getting students to stand in for the young people in the vehicle, using humour effectively to put the group at their ease. Grant, on the Peninsula, also moves comfortably around the stage, arranging the young people into the 'car', provoking friendly laughter as he light-heartedly and gently pushes the young men back into the car's 'boot'/trunk when they relax their pose during his description of the events. In another context Lawrence, from the Victoria Police Road Safety Education Unit – friendly, personable, but with the visible power and authority of the police officer – starts off with a story about his morning routine of calling into the office of the person whose job it is to update the road casualty statistics. With deceptive casualness he manages to convey a sense of urgency about the daily monitoring of road crash casualties. Towards the end of his presentation he invites a student up to address the group: 'If you were speaking to those people who have been involved in crashes overnight, what would you say to them?'

However, it is usually the (former) principal who, in conducting the introductory and plenary sessions, and providing the link for the workshop sessions throughout the day, acts as the main presenter and representative of the authority of Fit to Drive. The role carries a symbolic, as well as practical, function that is attached to their broader place within public culture. The former school principals who have joined the program as local area coordinators display/perform a particular style and conduct, the characteristic 'presence' of the principal/head teacher. The ease with which they speak with authority to large gatherings of students in the institutional setting of the school, or negotiate the world of bureaucracy and the political landscape, reveals a level of experience and tacit knowledge (Polanyi 1983) gained over many years in the role of principal. A common characteristic of many of these presentations is their manner of relating to young people, a way of establishing an immediate interest in their lives and careers. There is also a ready mutual recognition when speaking to other principal groups; the exchange of information, and signalling of shared knowledge and experiences. A distinct set of characteristics allows them to recognise each other and readily connect. There is a particular political benefit to be derived from the ease with which a former principal enters the spaces that form parts of the community of Fit to Drive. For example, Graham and other local area coordinators (LACs) have been invited to regional meetings of Catholic and other non-government school principals to speak about Fit to Drive. As former principals, they can 'talk the talk', appreciate the difficulties associated with taking the better part of a school day in senior school, and yet convince these groups of the benefits of participating in Fit to Drive.

The different moral authority embodied in the local area coordinator-as-former-principal can be understood in terms of Alasdair MacIntyre's (1981) description of certain 'characters' that figure in the moral and social landscape of our culture. These 'character' types are widely and easily recognisable in the cultural and institutional spaces they move in:

> There is a type of dramatic tradition – Japanese Noh plays and English medieval morality plays are examples – which possess a set of stock characters immediately recognisable to the audience. Such characters partially define the possibilities of plot and action. To understand them is to be provided with a means of interpreting the behaviour of the actors who play them, just because a similar understanding informs the intentions of the actors themselves; and other actors may define their parts with reference to these central characters. So it is with certain kinds of social role specific to certain particular cultures. They furnish recognisable characters and the ability to recognise them is socially crucial because a knowledge of the character provides an interpretation of the actions of those individuals who have assumed the character. It does so precisely because those individuals have used the very same knowledge to guide and to structure their behaviour.
>
> (MacIntyre 1981, p. 26)

These 'characters' differ from other, perhaps more publicly visible groups who have a particular role in society. It might be argued that they operate under the radar of public scrutiny and opinion that exists in relation to, for example, police. MacIntyre (1981) cites the example of the English school Headmaster (along with the Professor in Germany) as examples of what he means by 'character'. Characters, such as the Headmaster, were not just social roles, argues MacIntyre (1981, p. 28), but 'provided the moral focus for a whole cluster of attitudes and activities. They were able to discharge this function precisely because they incorporated moral and metaphysical theories and claims'. These theories and claims 'had a certain degree of complexity' and philosophical and professional differences and disagreements may exist within this group. MacIntyre (1981, p. 28) argues that this doesn't change the fact of the existence of a definable group representing the attributes of a recognisable character, who 'fused role with personal style, represented a moral and authority position recognised within the social and cultural milieu, and provided the culture with its moral definition'. When Graham says, 'I'm a former school principal – and don't I look it!' he is drawing on a fund of shared experience and assumptions about what that role might entail.

MacIntyre (1981) notes that, though the specifics of the role changes, the idea of the particular 'character' remains. If there are philosophical and professional differences regarding the nature of the principal, for example, the principal as entrepreneur, the 'idea' of principal remains strong, entrenched. A case in point is the expectation that the principal will be consistently present, visible, on the school campus; that they will know all the students by name, as far as possible; be the first at the 'front line' of any conflict or trouble; exercise moral authority; and 'set the tone' of the school with their very personality and character. This has been an important theme in the stories of Fit to Drive. The experience of so many of the former principals has been the role that they have been expected to play when road trauma has impacted on the school community.

Mobilising for the good?

> It has taught and made me aware of the risks, choices, responsibilities and impacts of my actions.
>
> (Female student, Rosehill Secondary College)

> Peer pressure can be a positive influence.
>
> (Male student, Sunnyside Secondary College)

A student from Rosehill Secondary College recommended the Fit to Drive workshop 'because it really opens people's eyes and gets friends talking about it'. What will the young woman and her friends be talking about? What is the 'frame' through which they will view the issue of road safety? Road safety promotion is inevitably associated with an awareness of the 'bad'. The news story we introduced at the beginning of this book described a crash that represents one of the worst possible scenarios that can play out in the fears of adults, lurking in their minds as an ever-present menace in the lives of young people. We described road safety efforts as being largely a process of mapping backwards, to understand causes of crashes; and forwards, to use that understanding in order to prevent future tragedies. Forensic analysis of road crashes, epidemiological studies of crash data, and behavioural research all contribute to the development of bodies of knowledge relating to road crash prevention. Road safety education often draws on disturbing examples and stories to distil lessons and develop messages for young people, and is concerned with, 'avoiding a bad' (James 2010). The student's feedback comment was written immediately following the screening of the short film that finishes the morning workshop. That film depicts a young man in a cemetery, talking to his friend, who had been killed in a car the young man was driving. 'Why did you let me speed?' he asks despairingly, as he limps away. The film is a reinforcement of the disastrous consequences of 'the bad' – speeding, negative peer pressure, irresponsibility.

Philosophically, Fit to Drive is aligned with James' pedagogical approach that appeals to the notion of teaching students to act 'under the notion of a good'. In the context of Fit to Drive this approach encompasses ideas of responsibility, restraint and care for others. The MFB case study, for instance, moves young people away from the notion of 'blame', to the idea of 'responsibility' as a positive 'good' (a moral imperative picked up by many of the student feedback responses). It promotes the idea that young people are capable (more capable than past generations) of finding solutions to the problem of road trauma. This emphasis on the 'good' is often overshadowed by the reminders of the 'bad' – grim consequences of crashes, and the negative behaviours associated with crash events. Nevertheless, the positive focus on young people's capacity for positive action (good) is asserted in the program's philosophy, expressed in statements such as 'young people have the answers' and 'young people taking responsibility'. The philosophy is evident in the efforts to engage young people's 'ownership' through the peer education focus, as well as the organisation of youth forums and initiatives to promote road safety in local communities. The assumption is that, if they are given the opportunity, and the encouragement, young people will – individually and/or within the group – develop positive values and make safe choices. This position is predicated on the understanding that young people are self-determining beings, able to exercise judgement and choice, not deterministically subject to impulsive, irrational behaviour. The notion of 'spreading the word' and influencing others – an idea taken up in many of the student feedback comments – connects with the ultimate aim of Fit to Drive: to contribute to building a culture of road safety within the community, beginning with family and friends. The intention conveyed in the statement of a 16-year-old female student (Devon Park Secondary College), 'I hope to go home and tell others/family about this', is echoed in many student feedback comments.

In our description of the early mobilisation of school principals around the prevention of young driver crashes we noted the resonances with other campaigns against perceived social harms, such as the 'war on drugs'. As an observer of the destructive human impulses that manifest in war, William James was interested in the idea of substituting positive ideals and pursuits for what he saw as innate military instincts in the human spirit. Suggesting that we need a 'moral equivalent of war', James (2010) was an early proponent of the harnessing of populations (particularly young people) in relation to positive projects and ideals. As Robert Richardson (2010, p. 12) notes in his introduction to a collection of James' essays, the modern 'war on drugs' may be an expression of those ideas – albeit with a focus on 'avoiding what is bad', rather than promoting a 'good'. While Richardson has highlighted the connections of James' ideas with modern manifestations of moral mobilisations, or 'wars', it is James' conception of educating for the 'good', as opposed to educating *against the 'bad'* that most accurately speaks to what the Fit to Drive program is aiming to do in its approach. As James (2010, p. xviii) argues,

> Spinoza long ago wrote in his *Ethics* that anything that a man can avoid under the notion that it is a bad he may also avoid under the notion that something else is good. He who acts *sub specie mali*, under the negative notion, the notion of the bad, is called a slave by Spinoza. To him who acts make freemen of your pupils by habituating them to act, wherever possible, under the notion of a good. Get them to habitually tell the truth. Not so much through showing them the wickedness of lying as by arousing enthusiasm for honour and veracity.

This acting 'under the notion of a good' is, further, dependent on our capacity to think (well), and to make the proper effort of attention:

> If, then, you are asked, '*In what does a moral act consist* when reduced to its simplest and most elementary form?' you can make only one reply. You can say *that it consists in the effort of attention by which we hold fast to an idea* which but for that effort of attention would be driven out of the mind by the other psychological tendencies that are there. *To think*, in short, is the secret of will, just as it is the secret of memory.

For James (James 1899, p. 94), discouragement of 'the bad' should be enacted through the substitution of 'positive' ideas, ideals and habits; the 'stock of ideas' that we have cultivated, the character that we have formed, will guide our action. 'Our moral effort, properly so called, terminates in our holding fast to the appropriate idea' (James 1899, p. 92). The benefits of this approach are to be seen, James argues, not only in its efficacy in preventing the 'bad'/ promoting the 'good', but also, in the long term effect of building character.

Fit to Drive, in taking up the practices and insights of health promotion and moral education, is concerned with not only reducing driving-related risks. It is also aware of the need to build positive values and promote positive environments, including a community of shared values in relation to road safety, which support young people in making safe choices. This involves making meanings that affirm personal safety and care for others, skills to (enact) the safe choices, and an environment that supports this. All of these involve acting for the notion of a 'Good'. The problematic nature of the 'Good' is something that we will return to at various times in what follows.

Notes

1 The next part of this section draws on Pike and Kelly (2014, pp. 102–106).
2 Our discussion here pre-empts a number of points that we will discuss and develop in greater detail in Chapter 6.
3 The RACV's young driver initiative 'Free to Go' became part of the program's 'show bag' promotion in 2009.
4 We discuss the Monavale story in greater detail in Chapter 6.

2 Rationality and risk

Limits and possibilities

Breath and the horror of the mundane[1]

Tim Winton's award winning 2008 novel *Breath* is an allegorical tale about the terror, for some young people, of being ordinary, and the ways in which surfing, sex and drugs provide the means for the story's main characters, Pikelet, Loonie, Sando and Eva, to identify, confront and challenge the limits shaped by this terror – sometimes with damaging consequences. In this tale the teenage years are imagined and experienced as being a time in a life in which the fear – the horror – of being ordinary compels Pikelet and Loonie to seek out, sometimes stumble upon, and embrace that which promises to make theirs *a life less ordinary*. In Winton's narrative a middle-aged Bruce Pike (Pikelet) explores his memories of a time in his life when he became entangled in a range of highly consequential behaviours and practices through a complex (damaging) series of relationships with the older, ex-champion surfer Sando and his (damaged) partner Eva. In these recollections risk, danger and harm – to be found, possibly, in increasingly reckless surfing adventures, drug use and sexual experimentation – are far from being things to be rationally calculated, or prudently managed with a wary eye to future consequences. Rather, they *breathe* energy, excitement, meaning and purpose into lifeworlds that, for Pikelet and Loonie, are dominated by the (imagined) institutionalised ordinariness of family, school and work in the relative isolation of the small, rural, working-class town of Sawyer on the southern coast of Western Australia. There is much in this tale that can move us towards the limits and possibilities of thinking about the roles that 'risk' plays in making some sense of what it is to *be* young.

In *Breath* risk and danger can be felt and experienced in ways that heighten the experience of being alive, of drawing breath. For many, the institutionalised ordinariness of everyday lifeworlds weighs heavily on what it means to live a life. For Pikelet and Loonie the mundane, ordinary limits of a life shaped by dominant, in some settings almost *frozen*, understandings of masculinity/femininity, age, family, school and work are things that can be challenged by the experiences to be found at the limits of skill and understanding that are promised first by surfing, then by drugs and sex. Yet, for many of Pikelet and

Loonie's peers, as Winton powerfully illustrates, these limit experiences are to be avoided (not even imagined). In this sense the ways in which Pikelet and Loonie embrace that which promises to make them, their lives, less ordinary are things that are not necessarily generalisable or translatable into the thinking and actions of their peers or, indeed, into the adults and adult institutions that shape their (young) lifeworlds. Pikelet's parents, like many adults in the contexts created by Winton, appear to have embraced the mundane and the ordinary as a means to account for the costs that can be associated with life's perils – to be found in Sawyer, in the ocean, the bush or the workplace.

It is a *steadiness* – the ordinariness that is characteristic of the institutionalised, adult environments of work, of marriage and relationships, of a daily life that is attractive or desirable because it is routine, dependable – that threatens to suck the breath out of life for Pikelet and Loonie.

In this account risk and danger, and what these might mean and the possibilities they provoke, the limits they transgress, are not always generalisable across time and space: they may, indeed, be situated in very particular configurations of time, space and place. To a middle aged man exploring his memories they are things that look very different from the ways they appear from the standpoint of a young man struggling against what is seen to be the monotony, the sheer ordinariness of breathing. Risk and danger can be easily, accidentally stumbled into; embraced out of emotions (embodied feelings) as diverse as fear or joy; rationally and prudently identified, weighed up and calculated (*or not!*) in situations and relationships which have a range of characteristics. These may be dependent, peer-based, characterised by bravado, shaped by masculinity and femininity, provoked by a need to belong, a desire to feel alive, a hunger not to be – a horror of being – *ordinary*. For example, when Pikelet, Sando and Loonie attempt to surf a massive, un-surfed, offshore break called Nautilus, Pikelet, unlike Sando and Loonie, cannot summon the courage to take on the ugly wall of water. After their first conquest of Nautilus, Loonie and Sando hatched plans to do it again, plans that excluded Pikelet. In the next few months a gulf opens between Pikelet and the other two, a gulf that sees Sando take the slightly older Loonie with him on a surfing trip to Java. This gulf and absence opens a space in which a potentially risky, dangerous sexual relationship can develop between Pikelet and Eva. Boredom, loneliness, listlessness and feelings of ordinariness conspire to send Pikelet out to the house after Sando and Loonie have left for Java. Winton tells a story of how a somewhat predatory and, possibly, spiteful, but more likely lonely and abandoned Eva, seduces an inexperienced, inept, fumbling Pikelet.

The act of drawing breath, the process of breathing and the consequences of not, are combined with the horror of ordinariness, the need to find and embrace that which marks one as not being ordinary, in the life that Winton breathes into Pikelet. The banality, the sheer ordinariness of breathing, takes on new dimensions when the sexual relationship between Pikelet and Eva evolves into Pikelet's introduction to Eva's auto-erotic asphyxiation fetishes.

While we are left to guess at much about the role of these fetishes in Eva's life we can imagine their connections (conscious or otherwise) to her craving for the danger, the fear, the risk to be found at the limits of life itself, at the limits of drawing breath. This uncertainty, ambiguity and risk profoundly scares Pikelet, but he is drawn into Eva's dangerous desires despite himself. The consequences for Pikelet of his stumbling into these fetishistic practices are immediate, but also echo throughout his life. These echoes give structure to Winton's narrative. The unfolding story leads us to the spaces in which a middle aged man reflects on a life that is profoundly shaped by consequences not imagined in the moments when he felt really alive at certain times in his youth.

Winton's novels – including *Cloudstreet* (1991), *The Riders* (1994), *Dirt Music* (2001) and *Breath* (2008) – are international best sellers and award winners. One reviewer of *Breath* hints at the appeal of these stories: '*His work is preoccupied with wounded or troubled characters, often haunted by their past, who set out on actual or psychological journeys in search of purpose, meaning and redemption*' (McDonald 2008, p. 19, our emphasis). These themes are not unique to Winton's work, and his appeal is not universal. But his sensibilities, his rhythms, his language, and the landscapes (material, symbolic, psychological) that his characters inhabit and are shaped by, speak powerfully to a sense of self, of place, of time, of human failings, limits and possibilities. He readily reaches into what might be called a soul to reveal truths about things that constitute the human condition. In spite of his popularity and critical acclaim these truths do not speak to all. They also do not answer to social scientific ways of understanding, describing, analysing, or generalising what it is to be human. But they are powerful on their own terms, especially as allegory. As another reviewer of *Breath* suggests: '*Who would have thought that a novel about an extreme sport, surfing the wild swells and sets off the south-western coast of Australia, would be about nothing less than the infirm glory of the human condition and the damage left in the wake of tasting the limits set for our human frame?*' (Mukherjee 2008, our emphasis).

But why is *Breath*, at many levels an allegorical tale, here? In this space? As we discussed earlier, much of what interests us in relation to understanding school based health promotion are the shifting relationships between what is made variously present, manifestly absent, and absent as Other. What might be the differing limits and possibilities of health promotion if the relationships between what is present, what is manifestly absent, and what is absent as Other shifted? What, if anything, would look different if risk, rationality and reason encountered the aesthetic in a troubling movement between the present, the manifestly absent, and the absent as Other?

So, in this chapter we want to explore some of the limits and possibilities of the ways in which understandings of 'risk', 'risk taking', and 'at risk' inform and shape the discourse of young people, road use and a whole array of concerns with young people's diverse behaviours and dispositions. In this work we seek to identify and make problematic the limits and possibilities of imagining young people's health and well-being in terms of risk, of devising and deploying health promotion interventions on the basis of risk discourses and rationalities.

The Fit to Drive workshop incorporates a large group presentation by a police officer, the rationale for which is to 'provide factual evidence about why young people are at risk on the road and how they can be safer road users' (Spence et al. 2006). This statement signals the key themes of rationality – the adoption of 'safe behaviours' through knowledge of 'facts' – and the mobilisation of risk discourses through which these facts will be interpreted and enacted. At many levels the program can be seen as sitting within the tradition of professional, expert, interventions that seek to help young risk takers to 'see the error of their ways and to adopt more "rational" behaviours' (Mitchell et al. 2004, p. 4). However, what is largely absent from this presentation of the 'facts' – an absence that our reading of *Breath* gestures towards – is any acknowledgement of the pleasures of driving, the aesthetics associated with driving practices and cultures. There is no discussion or acknowledgement of the aesthetic and erotic appeal of cars, the sensory pleasures of driving, nor of the symbolic and cultural significance of the car in contemporary life – what we will call the human-car-machine assemblage. The focus is on the car, and driving, as a potential source of danger. The absence of aesthetics/erotics/pleasure from health promotion discourses and interventions has been identified as a limit to promoting behaviour change with young people (Harrison et al. 2011). It is a limit we will find and test in what follows.

'Cold, hard facts'

Linda first provides some of her background, explaining that she is based at the nearby police station. She has experience of both the 'on road stuff' and education and community liaison as a youth resource officer. When it comes to road safety, she says, 'I can't make decisions for you. At the end of the day it's your decision, it's your choice.' This is in fact the slogan on the title slide of the police presentation. 'So basically what it's about today is you guys making the choice for yourself. There are consequences to doing the wrong thing on the roads. So, you make that decision, and you have to live with it. You can't put the blame on anyone else.'

Linda begins by raising the topic of 'distractions on the road' and asks the group for examples of distractions. Individual students are quick to respond: 'Car crashes'. 'Passengers'. 'Other motorists'. Some suggestions draw laughter and Linda re-frames these. 'Things that people do on the road, including people driving fast. What else? 'Cyclists …' She explores this further, then turns to the slide on the screen. 'So, there are some basic statistics for the state of Victoria.' She highlights some of the statistics on the screen: 'Every five minutes someone is injured on the roads. Every four days someone gets brain damage. And the one at the bottom … Every day someone dies. So today, in Victoria, someone will die from a road crash.'

The next slide appears, showing a graph depicting the crash profile of new drivers, including learner drivers. 'This graph shows that our learner drivers are the safest drivers on the roads. How many of you have got your Ls? Great, you guys are the safest drivers on the roads. How many have got your Ps? OK, not quite yet. Next year you will. As you can see, on the graph, there's learner drivers. Why do you think they're the safest?' A couple of the students respond. Linda repeats what they've said: 'Yes, because they have a responsible driver with them, teaching them …'

'So, high risk behaviour', Linda asks the group, 'what does that include?' As she picks up the ideas coming from the students the next slide comes up, depicting a still from a video: a head shot of a young man, dressed in a familiar football jumper. This is David Hille, a prominent player with the Essendon AFL football club. [2] *He is speaking to the camera: 'Yeah, myself and a group of friends, we felt a bit bored on the weekend, on a Saturday afternoon, and we thought we'd go for a skate. One of my friend's parents were away, and the car was there, and he got the keys, and, ah, we thought we'd take the car, and go and pick up a few friends and go to the local school and have a skate. Once we got to our friend's place, the school was only a kilometre away … By that time we'd lost control of the car and three of my friends had died. At the time you think perhaps you're a good driver. It just goes to show you're not at all. You don't have the experience that you require, and we weren't even fully licensed drivers, so … it was a risk from that point of view'.*

'I was in the front passenger seat, and I was lucky enough to get that seat because I was the tallest and the guys let me have the leg room. But that's the difference between, um, you know, being alive today, or not. We weren't really thinking at the time. It was a choice that came up, and I didn't really think about it. The driver lost control, and the people in the vehicle, it just kept … it came in contact with a tree, and ah … tore the car pretty much in half.'

As the film finishes, Linda addresses the group: 'So, do you know who he is?' The students recognise the footballer, and name him. 'He was very lucky to be alive' says Linda seriously. 'So if you remember from that video, he actually said that he got in the front seat because his legs were a little longer, and also … he made the choice to get in the car.' Linda discusses the role of peer pressure in these situations, and reflects on the lasting impact of the crash. 'Apparently that took him a long time to heal … Very emotional. If you can imagine being the one to survive a crash like that, three of your friends being killed. So that's pretty traumatic for him. He'll have to live with that for the rest of his life.'

'OK.' Linda turns to the next slide, which poses the question: 'What puts young people at risk on the roads?' Turning to the group she asks: 'Why do you think young drivers are at risk?' Scattered answers come from the audience, and picking up on one, she explores the issue of 'Inexperience'. 'You don't have that experience, but you'll get there.' The accompanying slide has a list of factors: inexperience, speed, overconfidence, lifestyle – alcohol, peer passengers, time of day, etc. 'We've worked out it's not good to have lots of people in the car at once,' observes Linda, 'Easily distracted. Overconfidence.'

The following slides depict a comparative graph of increased stopping distances with higher speeds, then increased injury severity and fatality risk with higher speeds on impact.

Other slides depict dangerous road conditions – fog, rain, gravel roads. They warn about the dangers of driving under the influence of alcohol, showing a statistical picture of the increased risk of crashing associated with different blood alcohol concentration levels.

Linda speaks to the next slides, which show information relating to the impact of alcohol, illicit drugs, fatigue and mobile phone use on driving – all measured in statistical terms. She is getting signals from the logistics coordinator that she needs to be finishing up – the recess bell will soon ring.

'So you guys have the right to tell the driver "no", if they're driving dangerously.' (This is reinforced by an image depicting a young woman with her hand outstretched, as in a 'stop' signal, assertively saying 'no'.)

The final slide has the closing message: 'Your life, your choice'. 'You guys know the consequences', says Linda, 'you know the law, so it's up to you'. With a final 'take care' she finishes up and hands over to the logistics coordinator. (Parkstone Secondary College, October 2009. Second large group session)[3]

'Cold, hard facts' are the main currency of this segment, as signalled throughout the presentation by the police presenter. The implication, that the opinions and attitudes that people commonly hold about road safety are based on ignorance of the 'facts', is counter-balanced against the appeal to the young people's immanent status as 'experts', alluded to in the introductory session of the workshop. The answer – to the over-representation of young people in road crashes – lies in young people, in themselves, they have been told. Armed with the 'facts', and motivation to change behaviours, they will be 'road safety champions'. In this sense, the last line of the PowerPoint presentation ('Your life, your choice') could be interpreted as an individualised message, not in tune with the Fit to Drive message, which is seen to be about young people taking responsibility for others, as well as themselves – a collective responsibility.

The short interviews with young road crash victims suffering long-term physical disabilities and brain trauma, as well as an interview with the AFL footballer David Hille about his experiences as a survivor of one of the Peninsula crashes, reinforce the importance of stories for preparing the 'emotional ground' for the assimilation of factual information. However, the road safety facts, and the associated messages delivered in this segment, are the main business of the session and are afforded an additional weight through the authority of the police. The police presence commands a distinct authority, even, or especially, among cohorts of young people where there is often an expression of resistance to police power.

The police officers possess different styles and levels of facility when delivering this presentation. Most aim for a relaxed, friendly approach, with the occasional joke. Some adopt a non-judgemental attitude (for example, in relation to illegal drugs and driving). Some are more engaging and interactive than others, often getting young people up from the audience to workshop safe messages to the audience. All, however, adopt a sober tone when talking about road crash risks.

The Power Point presentation emphasises facts and statistics relating to young people's involvement in road crashes, and to various aspects of road safety and crash risk: for example, statistics related to young fatalities and serious injuries. There is a particular focus on speed, alcohol and marijuana use, fatigue, distractions, and their impact on driving. Much of this information is framed in terms of increased risk associated with various activities and states, for example fatigue and crash risk. Crash risk after seventeen hours without sleep, the students are informed, is calculated to be equivalent to the crash risk of driving with .05 BAC. What is the significance of this roll-call of facts, and how is it used to construct the story about young people and driving?

'That won't happen to me' is the title of the leading slide in the presentation, a familiar statement that attempts to place in relief, and thus challenge, the indifference, denial, even illusion, that is perceived by road safety promoters to be a major impediment to motivating people to change their driving behaviours. Road safety messages are aimed at convincing young drivers that 'risky driving behaviours are in fact risky' (Imberger et al. 2011, p. 1). Statistics are used to construct an argument that aims to convince the young people that involvement in a road crash is a real possibility, and that the consequences will be serious: 'Every 30 minutes someone is injured, every four days someone becomes severely brain damaged, every 17 days someone becomes a paraplegic or quadriplegic, every day someone dies.' The relentless roll-call of statistics reinforces this point.

Young people and road safety: a health promotion problem made known through risk

Academic and policy understandings of road crashes and their prevention mostly mobilise discourses of 'risk' to analyse, explain, and develop policy in relation to road safety. Grounded in epidemiological methods, road crash analyses identify clusters of variables associated with incidence of road trauma to explain road crash prevalence, characteristics and, thus, causes. These variables are commonly identified as 'crash risk/s' (Senserrick and Haworth 2004; Toroyan and Peden 2007; Vassallo et al. 2007; Williams 2003).

Certain driving conditions are associated with a higher likelihood of a crash occurrence, and are defined as 'risky situations' (McKnight and McKnight 2003, p. 3). These situations aren't confined to young drivers, but are present as 'risks' for all drivers. Some situations aren't specifically related to driving behaviour (for example driving at night, in poor weather conditions, or on dangerous roads). Other 'risky situations' are directly attributable to driving behaviours that impede judgement, hazard perception and reactions, such as driving under the influence of alcohol or other drugs, or while fatigued, or using a mobile phone while driving (Harrison 2006; Mallick et al. 2007). Young people, however, are understood to be particularly 'at risk' in relation to driving and road use. In road crash analysis, age becomes, of itself, a *risk factor*:

> As beginning drivers, teenagers lack driving skills and also lack experience in recognizing *risky situations*. They are also more willing than adults to take *risks* behind the wheel, such as speeding and not buckling up. This combination of immaturity, inexperience and *risk-taking behaviour* produces *high crash risks* for teenage drivers. Graduated driver licensing (GDL) addresses these factors by phasing in on-road driving, allowing beginners to get their initial driving experience under *lower-risk* conditions.
>
> (Hedlund et al. 2003, p. 107, emphasis added)

This accumulation of factors identified with 'risk' leads to the conclusion that: 'every P plate driver is *at risk*', according to one warning to parents of P-plate drivers: 'limiting P plate driving to *less risky driving situations* in the first 12 months will help to *reduce the risk* of being involved in a crash' (Whelan and Oxley 2007, p. 4).[4] Young drivers are at a *higher risk* due to 'exposure to *risk* (drive more often and for longer distances and at high crash risk times) and making unrealistic assessment of *risks*' (VicRoads 2005). Risk, in this context, essentially refers to the likelihood of a crash. 'Novice drivers', irrespective of the age the beginner driver gets their licence, have a higher rate of crashes when compared with fully licensed drivers. *However*, younger novice drivers crash more often than older novice drivers, and 16-year-old novice drivers, in those states where 16-year-olds can obtain their driving licence, have higher crash rates again than 18-year-old novice drivers (Australian Transport Safety Bureau 2004; Toroyan and Peden 2007).

In road safety research statistical representations of crash occurrence and characteristics are analysed to identify conditions under which there is deemed to be an increased likelihood of a crash, and the severity or consequences of a crash. Apart from the age of the driver, these variables may include time of day, presence of passengers, involvement of alcohol or other drugs, road conditions and type of crash, including single vehicle crashes, which are more common in young novice drivers than older cohorts (Mayhew et al. 2002). These figures suggest, for example, that a 16-year-old is nearly three times as likely to crash as an 18-year-old (Preusser 2003, p. 1). The presence of peer-age passengers in the car significantly increases the likelihood of a crash (VicRoads 2005, p. 12). Around 26 per cent of first year P-plate drivers involved in fatal crashes are carrying two or more passengers, despite the fact that only 9 per cent of their total driving involves driving with two or more passengers (Arrive Alive 2012). This 'likelihood' of an event occurring is translated into a 'risk' – in the most basic sense a 'weighing up' of the possibility of the event occurring, based on statistics.

Much of the higher crash 'risk' of young drivers can be attributed to inexperience, not only with the management of the multifarious task of operating a motor vehicle, but with knowledge, 'reading' and responding to complex road conditions and driving situations (Senserrick 2007; Ferguson et al. 2007). In Australia particular types of crashes are more common amongst young drivers – such as right hand turns into oncoming traffic at intersections or running off the road on freeways (Williams 2003). Indeed, 'inexperience' is cited in road safety literature as the over-riding factor in young driver crashes (Senserrick and Haworth 2004; Shope 2007). The police presentation slide titled 'Why are young drivers at risk?' lists 'limited experience and skill' as the first factor. Related to this is their 'underestimation of level of risk'. That is, young people don't have the experience to recognise, prepare for and respond to risky situations on the roads.

'High level of exposure to risk', the second explanation, refers to the tendency of young people to drive longer distances, and more often, at times that involve high crash risk, such as night time (Williams 2003). However, road user research also reveals that more young drivers are involved in the dangerous behaviours that often result in fatalities and injuries, such as driving at unsuitable speeds for the environment, not using seat belts, overcrowding in cars, and driving while fatigued or under the influence of alcohol and other drugs (Catchpole and Styles 2005). Various studies have attempted to identify factors associated with risky driving, including early childhood and adolescent characteristics and developmental traits (Shope et al. 2001; Bingham and Shope 2004; RACV/VicHealth 2005; Styles et al. 2005; Vassallo et al. 2007; Keating and Halpern-Felsher 2008; Vassallo et al. 2010), and co-occurrence with other problem behaviours and personality traits (Gullone and Moore 2000; Machin and Sankey 2008; Vassallo et al. 2007). Other research has focussed specifically on personality traits leading to risky driving behaviours (Jessor 1987; Jessor 1996; Jessor et al. 1997; Hatfield and Fernandes 2009) and psycho-social and socialisation factors that are understood to influence risk taking and risky driving (Bina et al. 2006; Abbott-Chapman et al. 2008; Parker et al. 2009).

Risk discourses have assumed a dominant role in meaning making in relation to an array of issues determining young people's health and well-being. Deborah Lupton (1999a, p. 3) charts the changes in meanings of risk over time, in a movement from the so-called 'pre-modern' to 'modern', noting that these changes occured in the context of shifts in thinking about threats, dangers, and potentially calamitous events that constantly shadowed daily life. In pre-modern times, magic, superstition and associated beliefs were the foundation for various practices and customs people employed to 'deal with, contain and prevent danger' and thus exercise some sense of control over a frightening, and unknown, future. In the early modern era 'risk' started to be used as an expression describing uncertainties about, for instance, the outcomes of maritime ventures due to the arbitrary occurrence of natural events. Risk became entwined with technologies and systems related to insurance calculations (Ewald 1991; Luhmann 1993), and continued to express a sense of future events as being determined by fate, nature or the will of God (Scott and Williams 1992, p. 3). Importantly, risk in this sense still 'excluded the idea of human fault and responsibility'(Lupton 1999a, p. 5). In the modern era 'risk' has become a common way of explaining, understanding and ordering the world, in both lay understandings and expert discourses. 'Modernity', explains Lupton (1999a, p. 6):

> depends upon the notion, emerging in the seventeenth century Enlightenment, that the key to human progress and social order is objective knowledge of the world through scientific exploration and rational thinking. It assumes that the social and natural worlds follow laws that may be measured, calculated and therefore predicted.

As an outcome of this orientation to knowing the world humans became implicated in the production of 'risk' (as danger), and simultaneously responsible for its prevention. With the overriding idea that risk is calculable – a concept that underpins the development of technologies of risk such as insurance and epidemiology – the world and its 'chaotic manifestations, its contingencies and uncertainties' came to be viewed as within the control of human intervention (Lupton 1999a, p. 6). Technical/objectivitistic definitions of risk – where risk is an objective hazard that can be measured in terms of probability and severity of outcome – are common across many domains of knowledge and are foundational to discourses and practices relating to the management of human activity (Zinn 2009, p. 5).

Grounded in this understanding of dangers and harms as potentially being a consequence of human action, the word 'risk' has gathered different meanings, but has retained a level of neutrality which might encompass connotations of 'good', as well as 'bad'. In areas of finance, for instance, something could be regarded as a 'good risk' if it was seen as offering good returns. By the late twentieth century, however, 'risk' had become overwhelmingly associated with 'danger', and to a lesser extent an expression of calculations of probability (see Douglas 1992).

'Risk' is now a widely applied, multifaceted term, used in different contexts to mean a variety of things, from dangers and threats that surround us, to choices and decisions that people make in their everyday lives, to novel ways of expressing concerns about the vulnerability and dangerousness of certain population groups (Bessant et al. 2003; Kelly 2003; Lupton 1999a). According to Zinn (2009, p. 4) modern meanings of risk encompass three categories of ideas: danger or hazard, calculation, and risk taking. Missing from this account is the notion of 'at risk' as a description of status: a common way of constructing individuals and groups as specifically vulnerable to harm – due to issues that may include social, family and/or age status – and demanding of specific interventions.

Among key social and cultural theorists writing about 'risk' in recent years there is general agreement that, in what is sometimes referred to as 'late' or 'high modernity', an awareness of 'risk' figures significantly in individual consciousness and culture. Zinn (2009, p. 2) argues that 'to interpret issues in terms of risk seems itself to be a particular way of viewing our world in terms of politics, science, or everyday life'. In *Risk Society*, Ulrich Beck (1992, p. 19) framed the question of risk as a fundamental feature of modern life by examining the impact of the constant menace of large-scale, uncontrollable – often invisible – risks threatening our environment and our health: 'in late modernity the world is perceived as a dangerous place in which we are constantly confronted with risk'. Beck's concept of 'risk society' encompasses the claim that the modern world contains risks that have never previously been encountered, which are, potentially, unmanageable, and that this gives rise in individuals to generalised anxiety, a sense of being out of control.

A risk society sensibility (Beck 1992) is also evident in discourses of driving and road use. In the minds of many people the driving environment is heavily laden with symbolism of hostile forces at work: the roads and freeways, the high-powered cars with their tinted windows, their loud, seemingly apocalyptic music, terrifying trucks, ordinary drivers who can suddenly transform into 'monsters in metal cocoons' (Lupton 1999b). In this frame these are real, looming, quasi-anonymous risks which have to be anticipated, calculated and even fatalistically accepted. Images of car crashes come to symbolise the arbitrary rule of death and the transitory nature of life: 'Statistics show that driving a car is one of the most dangerous things a young person will ever do.'[5] This threatening, doom laden view is counter-balanced by the positive symbolism represented in driving the car: being in control, mastery, possessing a personal domain, as well as a more benign relationship to the car and driving. We take up this point shortly.

Anthony Giddens (1991), like Beck (1992), is interested in the increasingly individualised nature of social biographies in 'late modernity'. From this perspective individuals are obliged to 'construct their own biographies' in an era of de-traditionalisation, and the destabilisation of the previously taken-for-granted social world. The unsettling of traditional social and community structures means that individuals are required to exercise 'lifestyle choices', to make decisions about their life-paths in the context of an ever-changing social (economic, technological) landscape. Giddens (1991, p. 5) maintains that risk constitutes a key way of thinking about life choices, when individuals are required to choose between a plethora of options and alternatives: 'The more tradition loses its hold … the more individuals are forced to negotiate lifestyle choices among a diversity of options'. Young people are imagined as being particularly exposed to the imperatives of individualised biographies at a time of 'globalised uncertainty' (Cebulla 2009, p. 40), and futures are imagined and constructed with a heightened awareness of risk. The conditions for this awareness have been created in the emergence of a pervasive 'risk culture' which Giddens (1991, p. 244) describes as 'a fundamental cultural aspect of modernity in which awareness of risk forms a medium of colonising the future'. However, the task of constructing individualised biographies is overshadowed by the uncertainty of outcomes of individual decisions in the context of increasing – and increasingly complex – social risks, and a lack of trust in systems of expert knowledges (Cebulla 2009; Lupton and Tulloch 1998, Taylor-Gooby and Zinn 2006). Moreoever, this increasing 'responsibilization of citizenry' (Kemshall 2008, p. 21) is a chimera when structural factors continue to constrain equitable access to options and choices (Furlong and Cartmel 1997; Kelly 2006).

Health is a key site of the reflexive project of the self, one that requires considerable personal commitment (Spruijt-Metz 1999). It is both an individual objective and a responsibility as a citizen: '[l]ike health, responsibility is a major value of the modern age, and in a way it is based on a philosophy of the Enlightenment. Responsibility means more autonomy, taking fate into one's own hands' (Beck-Gernsheim 2000, p. 131). Responsibility for health has increasingly been devolved to the individual. Scott and Williams (1992, p. 3) argue that the period since the 1970s has seen 'an *ideological shift* from the rights of individuals to have their health protected by the State, to the responsibilities of individuals to protect themselves from risk'. As Giddens (1991, p. 56) argues, to be judged a 'competent agent' one must be seen by others to be in control of our bodies, and, by extension, in control of our decisions and actions.

Young people and the problem of risk

The interest in young people and 'risk' is not confined to road safety. Since the 1980s concepts of 'risk' have become central to analysis and interventions relating to young people. Interpretations of young people 'at risk' shape public policy and underpin programs and interventions with young people. Some commentators contend that risk-based approaches are a manifestation of increased governance of young people and provide a pretext, within a familiar context of moral panic about youth, for the introduction of new ways of regulating this section of the population (Bessant et al. 2003; Hewitt et al. 2006; Tait 2000). Evidence of such regulation is to be found in interventions targeting young people such as crime prevention, drugs, health – particularly sexual health – education, homelessness, and driving and road use.

One of the motivating forces behind the interest in the study of risk, risk perceptions and risk behaviours is, suggest Mitchell et al. (2004, p. 1), the commitment to enhancing the health status of populations:

> in relation to youth in particular, one can identify a strand of research that derives from what might be said to be general efforts of modern societies to enhance the health and well-being of their populations and to exert increasing control over our lives and our environments.

Young people are seen as particularly vulnerable to an array of potential threats emanating from rapidly changing social conditions (Davis 1999), and the perceived disintegration of modern culture (Eckersley 1988, 1992). In this view, young people, as the 'social canaries' (Eckersley 2005) of a culture, are the first group to suffer, to display the symptoms caused by the ills of modern life.

Academic and professional concerns with issues of risk have tended to focus on two distinct but connected notions of risk: *risk taking* as a universal feature of adolescence on the one hand; and the identification of particular young people as being *at risk* on the other. Moreover, institutions and authorities concerned with the well-being and regulation of young people draw on research which identifies particular *risk factors* placing young people specifically *at risk* in given circumstances. Young people are described as 'at risk' due to a range of factors, for example homelessness, disrupted family lives, refugee background, and general social disadvantage (Chamberlain and Mackenzie 1998; Poynting and White 2004). The fields of adolescent health and welfare have seen the development of inventories of 'risk and protective factors' operating in young people's lives, and the creation of interventions based on this analysis. This analysis often collapses two distinct concepts into the term 'at risk': as a description of young people's vulnerable psycho-biological and social status in which *risk factors* indicate a cluster of variables such as loss of parent, disrupted family environment or living in a neglected neighbourhood. These risk factors predict *health-risk behaviours* (Hawkins et al. 1992; Hawkins et al. 1999). At the same time engagement in *high risk behaviour* is identified as a risk factor in itself.

These ideas connect with understandings of young people as *risk takers*, as well as young people *at risk* due to inherent characteristics – their inexperience, biological factors, lifestyle and peers. The term 'at risk' carries resonances of young people as either 'victims' or 'threats'. The concept of young people as 'risk takers' recalls ideas about adolescence as a period of turmoil and rebellion or 'storm and stress'[6] (Bessant et al. 1998; Jones 2009; Hall 1931; Muuss 1996). In this sense young people are said to be governed by the emotions caused by hormonal upheavals, and the adolescent body is imagined as 'unruly, uncontained, uncontrolled' (Lupton and Tulloch 1998). Risk taking is represented as usually, but not always, problematic. A certain degree of risk taking is sanctioned and deemed important for young people's maturation and self-esteem (Crisp 2010). Adolescence is imagined as 'a natural period of experimentation and risk-taking' (Plant 1992, p. 9). Risk taking is also seen to serve developmental functions: 'risk taking should be seen to have definite functions for the young related to their development and to the attainment of symbols that seem to confirm adult status' (Franzkoviak 1988, p. 43). In addtion, risk taking is conceived as being important to the everyday lives of young people (France 2000, p. 318). This idea is linked to an interpretation of adolescence, rooted in developmental psychology, which understands adolescence as involving the completion of specific psycho-social tasks (see for example Erikson 1971; Mooney 2000). These ideas are framed by assumptions about young people as being rebellious; as possessing a sense of personal invincibility; as being ignorant about, and lacking concern for, possible consequences of health-damaging behaviours; and as being particularly subject to peer group influence.

To a significant degree young peoples' vulnerability to danger and harm, to risk, is attributed to their own behaviours and choices. Risk perception is seen to be a key factor in young people's behavioural choices (for example in relation to drug use, sexual activity, personal safety, driving). As a consequence experts and professionals are interested in discovering how young people perceive and make judgements about risk, often highlighting a young person's 'decision-making competence' and 'risk taking *style*' (Millstein and Halpern-Felscher 2002).

Behavioural psychologists have developed different theories and models of risk to account for the 'risk' behaviours of young people. The health sciences have developed elaborate models of health and risk behaviours to account for individual choices and actions, including Social Cognitive Theory, the Health Belief Model, the Theory of Reasoned Action and Subjective Culture, Interpersonal Relations Theory, and Problem Behaviour Theory (Jessor 1991; Jessor and Jessor 1977; Arnett 1996; Horvath et al. 2012). These sorts of studies attempt to isolate the risk perceptions, risk judgements and risk behaviours of individuals and specific population groups. They cross-correlate predisposing determinants, social conditions and clusters of personal characteristics, to build a picture of particular cohorts of young people and their predisposition to taking specific risks, or risk taking in general (see for example Gullone and Moore 2000). Some areas of youth studies have drawn on these models from the psychological and health sciences literature to interpret young people's activities, culture and choices (see for example Plant 1992). Indeed, specific developmental traits have been linked to driving-related risk taking (Bingham and Shope 2004; Vassallo et al. 2007).

Tulloch and Lupton (2003, p. 1) highlight the limitations of theoretical approaches to risk perception that overlook the importance of the social and cultural milieu in shaping individual risk assessment, perceptions of danger and safety, and alternative action: 'understandings about risk, and therefore the ways in which risk is dealt with and experienced in everyday life, are inevitably developed through membership of cultures and subcultures as well as through personal experience'. In this sense, commonly cited distinctions in research and practice between 'voluntary' and 'involuntary' risks can be inaccurate and unhelpful. Highlighting the role played by 'unarticulated assumptions, moral values and practices in people's responses to risk', Tulloch and Lupton (2003, p. 6) argue that people respond to risk 'emotively and aethestically as members of cultural subgroups rather than as atomized individuals'. The emotional dimension is an important element of risk perception, not only in the heightened states of excitement, fear or distress, but in everyday risk assessment where 'emotions are used as a kind of advisor, referring to complex experiences which cannot be transformed in formalized objective knowledge' (Zinn 2009, p. 14). In this sense Scott Lash (1994) emphasises the aesthetic dimension of risk, which is reflexively embodied in the aesthetic practices of self-interpretation involving taste and style, consumption, leisure and popular cultures. Here, risk perception and assessment involves sophisticated processing of signs and symbols rather than simply the accumulation and assessment of 'information' and is closely linked to group identification and membership.

In addition, a body of work drawing on Foucault's work on governmentality and the care and practices of the self, suggests that neo-liberal governmentalities shape and mobilise discourses of risk, of youth at-risk, in attempts to manage the uncertainties of globalised, institutionalised risk environments – environments in which the practices and programs of welfare state liberalism are no longer imagined as being fit for purpose. The ideal self, as imagined by these arts of government, is able to imagine itself as an enterprise. This is a self that is autonomous, choice making, prudent, risk aware, and, above all, responsible. Such a form of selfhood, a view of what it is to be person, is embedded in many governmental programs in the neo-liberal democracies at the start of the twenty-first century. Of course this sort of self, as an ideal, is something that many of us, at different times, would struggle to embody. It is also a self, as imagined in these governmentalities, that needs to be encouraged – sometimes, incited, often compelled – to emerge. Through various programs, through education and training, in schools, on the job, elsewhere. Young selves, in this sense, are often imagined as being *at risk* of not developing these attributes, capabilities and comportments. Programs, interventions and practices need to be developed and deployed to encourage the young self to imagine itself as an enterprise, as being, potentially, autonomous, choice making, prudent, risk aware, and responsible (see Kelly 2013, 2011, 2007, 2006).

An emerging feature of risk-focussed understandings of young people is the burgeoning medical research into adolescent brain development, some of which claims to be able to identify certain characteristics of the adolescent brain that appear to predispose young people to risk taking (Sunstein 2008; O'Neill 2010), specifically driving-related risks (Reyna and Farley 2007; Dahl 2008). Although neuroscientists themselves advise caution when extrapolating from brain-imaging studies to interpretations and predictions of behaviour (Giedd et al. 1999; Giedd 2004; Steinberg 2008), 'teen brain' theories have been enthusiastically embraced by adolescent health specialists to explain young driver crashes (and to advocate for legislative restrictions, including curfews, on young drivers). For example, an article in a metropolitan newspaper in the wake of a dramatic crash resulting in the deaths of several young people cited academic psychologists referring to the adolescent brain as an explanation for '*the need for speed*' (Szego 2010). Populist writers often combine 'teen brain' explanations with old ideas about 'raging hormones' to portray young drivers as a lethal cocktail of sensation seeking, risk taking, 'loose cannons', incapable of reasoning and sound decision making (see for example Biddulph 2007; Carr-Gregg 2007; Bennett 2007): 'An immature brain, together with the hormones that stir them up and drive them to be thrill-seekers (especially for young men), is a potentially dangerous mix' (Bennett 2007). Michael Carr-Gregg (2007) believes the causal link is self-evident:

> Adolescents have significant neurological deficiencies that cause stark limitations of judgement … The general consensus among neuroscientists is that the maturation process is not completed until young adulthood: perhaps as late as 30 years of age, making the teenage brain inherently less capable of balancing emotions and more likely to exhibit risk-taking behaviour … The result of this delay in brain development can be seen clearly on the roads.
>
> (Carr-Gregg 2007)

Neuroscientific, or neurobiological (Sunstein 2008) explanations of 'risk taking behaviour' – which assume risk-taking as a universal feature of adolescence – have started to appear both in general youth policy as well as research underpinning youth health policy (Australian Institute of Health and Welfare 2011; Victorian Government Department of Human Services 2008). For example, references to 'teen brain' theories appear in young driver policy in Australia: 'evidence from studies examining brain maturation supports the notion that driving may be affected by the lack of maturation until late adolescence or beyond' (Australian Transport Council 2011, p. 82). Biddulph's (2007) article on the impact of neurological and other biological factors on young drivers was has been reproduced on the Transport Accident Commission (2015) road safety school resources website and the NSW *Youthsafe Newsletter* (Youthsafe 2006) featured an article on the link between neurobiological development and risk taking: '[r]ecent research from the field of neuroscience is shedding new light on the question of why teenagers engage in reckless risk taking behaviours'. While there is a recognition of the complex interplay of knowledge, culture, (in)experience and social norms in the mix of factors contributing to young driver crashes – the 'teen brain' explanation remains a seductive idea (Vick 2003, 2005). We will return to some of these concerns in Chapter 7 where we review a number of critiques of discourses of adolescent brain development (Bessant 2008; Kelly 2012; Sercombe (2010).

Interlude: the aesthetics and erotics of the human-car-machine assemblage

It is telling that the culturally symbolic significance of the car, with the associated imagery of machine, technology, power and speed, is afforded no sanctioned place in the cultural iconography of Fit to Drive. The potent and pervasive presence of the motor vehicle in our cultural imagination is never evoked in the workshop, though it forms a distinct part of the 'hinterland' (Law 2004) of Fit to Drive. There appears to be, in fact, a conscious distancing from this imagery. And yet the dominant 'idea' of the car, and its aesthetic and erotic dimensions, plays a significant role in shaping the context within which people approach the act of driving, of being in a motor vehicle, of the human-car-machine assemblage: 'the car is partly constitutive of who it is to be "us". The centrality of the motor car in our culture is both taken-for-granted and idealised' (Paterson 2007, p. 123).

> We affirm that the world's magnificence has been enriched by a new beauty: the beauty of speed. A racing car whose hood is adorned with great pipes, like serpents of explosive breath – a roaring car that seems to ride on grapeshot is more beautiful than the Victory of Samothrace.
>
> (Filippo Marinetti, *Futurist Manifesto* [1909/1972, p. 41])

> From time to time we sensed it, as we watched an express train thundering at lightening speed across the countryside, a race-car shooting into its lane from a banked curve, or screeching birds wheeling above our cities ... we sensed that some surplus lived and breathed there, a luxury, an excess of energy, a will to transform all of life into energy.
>
> (Ernst Jünger, 1919 [quoted in Theweleit 1996, p. 199])

With the previously unimagined possibilities offered by the modern motor car, speed becomes the enduring, strident doppelgänger of the utilitarian motor vehicle. The experience – and the even more intoxicating *idea* – of speed is embraced by car enthusiasts and conscripted into the service of particular world views. From its earliest appearance, some intellectuals, artists, writers and political activists saw in the car – supreme among machines – an expression of their philosophical ideas about life, human existence and the social world. As a symbol of the forces unleashed by the Machine Age, *speed* was adopted as a positive force, aesthetic ideal and object of desire by the Futurist movement in the first decades of the twentieth century. For the Futurists, who worshipped 'the beauty of speed', the car was the ultimate speed-machine, and speed represented the 'synthesis of every courage in action. Aggressive and war-like'. Speed brought possibilities of transcendence through immersion in the divine: 'the intoxication of great speed in cars is nothing but the joy of feeling oneself fused with the only *divinity*'. In contrast, slowness was equated with 'analysis of every stagnant prudence. Passive and pacifistic' (Marinetti 1916/1972, p. 95).

The life-force attributed to the machine was celebrated by the German writer Ernst Jünger. For Jünger machines were connected with Nietzsche's 'will to higher and deeper goals': 'Yes, the machine is beautiful; its beauty is self-evident to anyone who loves life in all its fullness and power' (Jünger 1922, quoted in Theweleit 1996, p. 197). Distinguishing between 'useful' and 'expressive' machines, Jünger argued that: 'The machine must be made more than a mere means of production to satisfy our pitiful needs; it should provide us with a higher, a deeper satisfaction' (ibid.).

This imagery of speed, machine and violence found an echo in the ideology, aesthetics and erotics of early twentieth-century fascism, with which significant elements of the Futurist movement were aligned. Associated with the machinery of war – recalling Marinetti's coupling of military imagery with descriptions of the car: 'a roaring car that seems to ride on grapeshot' – speed also became a central motif in the proto-fascist literature of post-World War I Germany, as Klaus Theweleit (1996) reveals in his study of the fascist psyche. Drawing on his analysis of novels and memoirs of the former imperial soldiers of the Freikorps, Theweleit argues that the emotional core of fascism is sustained by what Walter Benjamin called a 'technologically amplified aestheticism' expressed in the machine (Benjamin and Rabinbach 1996, p. xii). In the newly constituted relationships within this technological aesthetic, the object of desire becomes the merging of self with machine. The machine is to be used 'to resolve the problems of the body' (Theweleit 1996, p. 197), including the inconvenient drives and desires generated by the body. The fascist aesthetic is characterised, according to Theweleit, by 'the desire to rid themselves of their own tormenting feelings – the bodily stirrings that could never again be integrated once released' (Theweleit 1996, p. 348). Eros is denied, desire itself is sublimated in destructive action, and 'sexuality [is placed] at the service of destruction' (Benjamin and Rabinbach 1996, p. xiii).

The iconography of the fetishised motor vehicle, with its promise of extremes of speed – rendered so vividly by the Futurist/Fascist movement of the early twentieth century – has continued into the twenty-first century. It manifests in the consumer culture across many domains: advertising, media, film, video games and public entertainment presented as sport. The orgiastic rapture with which the purveyors of cars and speed-as-entertainment and life-force celebrate the driving 'experience', and the car-object, recalls the metallic, over-heated prose of the early twentieth-century Futurist writers.

This rapture is intimately connected with the promise of violence, the allure of pain. Marinetti (1909/1972, p. 40) likens cars to wild animals, invoking sacrificial images when he describes his attraction to 'the famished roar of automobiles'. Reverentially approaching the automobiles:

> We went up to the three snorting beasts, to lay amorous hands on their torrid breasts. I stretched out on my car like a corpse on its bier, but revived at once under the steering wheel, a guillotine blade that threatened my stomach.

There is a current of violence that shadows the human relationship to the motor car. It is a legacy born of the Futurist/Fascist aesthetic and ideology, which embraced the symbolism of the machine as instrument of war – a force for destruction rather than force for life. No fruitful, generative, playful cyborg hybrids here: 'In displaying the destructive potential of technology, war has transformed pleasure in technology into fear; it has further deepened the opposition between humanity and machinery' (Theweleit 1996, p. 201). The violence associated with the human-car-machine assemblage paradoxically perpetuates this opposition and justifies the fear.

The violence that resides at the core of the car culture has been explored by a number of writers. Violence visited on the communal space by the car's colonisation and eventual dominance of the landscape extends from the aggressive occupation of space (and time), and the generation of barely endurable levels of noise, through to the threat of physical violence caused by collisions (Urry 2007). It includes the threat, and acts, of violence generated by the human-car-machine assemblage engaged in acts of aggression (Lupton 1999b), and the violent sexualised male fantasies enacted within the car space, exploited, reproduced and created by automobile advertisers and other media (Jain 2006). The car as weapon is vividly present in modern consciousness (Paterson 2007).

The speeding human-car-machine assemblage is associated with a transformative, almost transcendental, energy. An assemblage that becomes 'a vehicle for the expression of carnal desire' (Theweleit 1996, p. 199). The supreme expression of this desire is found (sought) in war. But Theweleit reveals the cultural conditions and system of social relations that gave rise to the 'psychic compulsion which associates masculinity with hardness, destruction, and self-denial' (Benjamin and Rabinbach 1996, p. xiii), a set of values recognisable in other social, historical and contemporary settings. The cultural ideal of masculinity embedded in a set of attributes associated with hardness and violence, and the rejection of the 'feminine', recalls Allan Patience's (1992) description of the 'Hard Culture' at the heart of Australian social and cultural values. Patience (1992, p. 60) argues that the psyche, social relationships and bounded possibilities of identity formation and self-actualisation of the young Australian male cannot be understood outside the specific historical and cultural landscape of (white) Australian society. There is, he argues, a fundamental substrate of 'hard culture' values operating in (male) Australian culture, associated with aggression, violence, anti-intellectualism, and denial of the 'feminine' (see also Connell 2000). Pleasure in the power of the human-car-machine assemblage and speed is intrinsic to a male culture that pursues that which allows for the 'elimination of the feminine' (Kenway et al. 2006). Importantly, one of the ways this elimination of the feminine finds expression is in a celebration of motor vehicles and speed (Walker 1999; Graham and White 2007).

These values have found a comfortable home, and taken on a characteristic form, in the modern car culture. However, the supremacy of the motor car has been subject to resistance and critique. Since the development of the steam train and expansion of the railways there has been an expression of ambivalence in modern culture towards the motor vehicle. Dismay at the railroad's encroachment into the Arcadian landscape of the countryside (Gaskell 2000), or resentment of the car's intrusion into, and dominance of, modern life – 'such life as is conferred by the stench of motor-cars' (Forster 1989, p. 29) – are themes present in the novels of nineteenth- and early twentieth-century authors.

In the world of the 'aggressive, war-like' car, there appears to be an ever-shrinking place for the passive, unassuming, utilitarian, and slow, vehicle. This reality is poignantly depicted in Jacques Tati's hapless recreational car depicted in his dystopic 1971 film *Trafic* (Tati 2008), in which both driver (M. Hulot) and his car are victims of the relentless, unforgiving driving environment.

Ideas of speed, testing the power of cars and engines, using the car as a technology of dominance and extension of personal power, are representative of prevailing cultural values that feature in the expression of personal identity, particularly (though not exclusively) among many young males. Young people who may not necessarily share these values (at least to the degree of some of their peers) may still find themselves in situations where identification with these cultural and social values shapes the performance of identity in the form of recreational choices and behaviours. They may, in short, get caught up, against their inclination and judgement, in dangerous driving situations. The relationship to the car – embracing and/or rejection – is part of modern subjectivity.

Beyond rationality and risk?[7]

The presentation of road safety facts and messages in the police information session is grounded in dominant objectivist risk-based accounts of road crash analysis and road safety. The Fit to Drive program's employment of risk is aligned with discourses of calculative rationality and technologies of governance that construct complex human behaviour in terms of calculable and mediated risk. Rationality is engaged through the framework of risk. Meanings and interpretations of risk are complex, contested and constantly shifting. Socio-cultural perspectives on risk focus on the ways in which social, cultural and subcultural environments shape and influence subjective risk perceptions and responses.

If we return to our reading of Tim Winton's (2008) *Breath* we can read a tale that might not necessarily be *real*, but which may be profoundly *truthful* in terms of the ways in which it provokes us to imagine how some young people experience the limits and possibilities of the ordinariness and banality of everyday life: an ordinariness that emerges from, and shapes, the particular institutionalised lifeworlds of a remote, rural, working-class town on the southern coast of Australia. In *Breath* Winton enacts realities in which knowing something of young people and risk is *embodied*, is *emotional*, is *situated*, is *allegorical* (Law 2004). Part of the power of Winton's narrative is that it is a story told from the vantage point of middle age. From this standpoint – hindsight – we can selectively review a life and identify and locate missed opportunities, successes, failings, thwarted ambitions, unrealised dreams, unfulfilled fantasies. At the end of the story the middle aged Bruce Pike reflects on a life marked by personal loss, a broken marriage, physical and mental breakdown, and some sort of parlous redemption. Winton's use of hindsight, of memory, provides Bruce Pike with the opportunity to reflect on and reconstruct a past with a certain worldliness, an insightfulness, a sense of opportunities – lost and taken. As a technique that enables *Breath* to work as allegory, *hindsight* provides us with a vantage point that we don't possess in the now, in the moments when we choose, embrace, stumble upon things that may be far reaching in consequence and significance – when we are young and/or old. Yet, as we have seen, so much of social/behavioural science, policy and service delivery discussions construct risky practices in ways that suggest that current generations of young people ought have developed a risk aware, prudent, responsible disposition to present practices and future consequences. Ought to be able, with *foresight*, to imagine and colonise their futures in ways that can guard against damage, hurt and pain. To, in effect, dis-enchant their presents and futures. To render them amenable to calculation, guided by expertise, informed by evidence.

John Law (2004, p. 92) argues that in our everyday, sense-making existence we are all – expert and non-expert, scientist and artist – 'allegorists'. We 'read between the lines and manifest realities that are not being spoken about in as many words'. We unsettle, interfere with the 'boundaries between that which is Othered and that which is manifest'. In this way we can imagine that as allegorists we are, much of the time, 'crafting and manifesting realities that are non-coherent, that are difficult to fit together into a single smooth reality'. The promise of allegory is that it can make us less certain of what we think we know about young people and risk. This uncertainty might provoke us to explore how those things that are absent, Othered, impossible might contribute to our understanding if they could be imagined as possible. *Breath*, in itself, has its own limits. The roles that such allegorical tales may play in shaping accounts of young people and risk are dependent on the associations that they can establish, the meaningfulness that they can add, to other ways of knowing young people and risk (Clifford 1986). When we do social science we become literalists. We employ knowledge practices that aim for, and gain credence from, a capacity to describe, analyse and represent things directly, truthfully. The particular power of *Breath* is that it is an allegorical tale that is situated, embodied and told from the vantage point of hindsight. A tale told from the vantage point of hindsight can be a powerful vehicle for unsettling what it is that the social and behavioural sciences can tell us about youth (as becoming) and risk (as mitigated by prudential foresight). The tales told in *Breath* can situate an array of what we might imagine as risky practices in an always uncertain relationship to particular emotional, psychological and cultural responses to the horror of being ordinary – whatever that might mean in the diverse institutionalised lifeworlds that shape young people's lives.

How far the truths of this tale about surfing, about growing up in relative remoteness and isolation, about the horror of ordinariness, travel from these spaces is something that can't be determined by this reading. At this point we want to draw a provisional line under this discussion with what English critic James Wood (2008, pp. 178–179) suggests we might find if we go looking for meaning and knowledge in practices other than the ones we are often encouraged, even compelled, to use in the practice of twenty-first-century social science. He argues that: 'the question of fiction's referentiality – does fiction make true statements about the world? – is the wrong one, because fiction does not ask us to *believe* things (in a philosophical sense) but to *imagine* them (in an artistic sense)'. In this sense, imagining 'the heat of the sun on your back is about as different an activity as can be from believing that tomorrow it will be sunny. One experience is all but sensual, the other wholly abstract'.

This sense of imagination provides a means to move beyond the problematic arena of *reality*, to a sometimes more problematic notion of *truth*. If, as Wood (2008, p. 180), suggests we 'throw the term "realism" overboard, we can account for the ways in which, say, Kafka's *Metamorphosis* and Hamsun's *Hunger* and Beckett's *Endgame* are not representations of likely or typical human activity, but are nevertheless harrowingly truthful texts'. In truth, if not in reality, we can imagine 'what it would feel like to be outcast from one's family, like an insect (Kafka), or a young madman (Hamsun), or an aged parent kept in a bin and fed pap (Beckett)'.

And so as we encounter a variety of texts and representations we can stumble upon what Wood (2008: p. 184) calls the 'blue river of truth': the space in which we might engage 'scenes and moments and perfectly placed words in fiction and poetry, in film and drama, which strike us with their truth, which move and sustain us, which shake habit's house to its foundations'. It is in these moments, in these encounters with the likes of Pikelet and Eva, that we might realise the potential for understanding what it means to be human that is promised by Mills' *sociological imagination*, but which is oftentimes thwarted by the governmentalised knowledge practices that characterise the social sciences at the start of the twenty-first century.

It is these moments, from these experiences and experiments, that we might also think differently about the limits and possibilities of making the problems of young people and health promotion knowable and governable in terms of reason, risk and rationality. In doing so we would stress again that reason, risk and rationality are not wrong (headed), nor that they have no useful place in what we might call a critical encounter with the diverse problems of young people and health promotion. The challenge we take up here is how embodied meaning making, pleasures and pain, aesthetics, can add productive dimensions to the troubling of the limits and possibilities of reason, risk and rationality. How the aesthetics and erotics of the human-car-machine assemblage, most often absent as Other, even manifestly absent from concerns about young people, road safety and risk, enable us to imagine possibilities beyond these limits.

Notes

1 This opening section draws on work first published in Kelly (2011).
2 Australian Football League.
3 Parkstone is a government all-girls school in Melbourne's north, where the police presenter, 'Linda', is one of the local police youth resource officers.
4 'P plate' refers to probationary drivers. In the current Victorian graduated licensing system, provisions drivers are subject to driving restrictions according to the length of time they have had their licence.
5 The (then) Victorian state government minister for transport, Peter Batchelor (VicRoads 2005, p. 3).
6 The term 'storm and stress' derives from the eighteenth-century German literary movement (*Sturm und Drang*) which was associated with rebellious and volatile youth. It was subsequently coined to characterise the life stage of adolescence.
7 This section draws on arguments first presented in Kelly (2011).

3 Engaging emotions, exploring values, mobilising rationality

'A moment of emotional truth …'

Burton Secondary College, a school in Melbourne's inner-north, is one of those outer-suburban schools that suffered a poor reputation until recently, when it has been attracting more of a mix of students from middle-class, educated families as well as the traditional cohort of young people from the established working-class community surrounding the school. The workshop is taking place in the school hall, with its drab flat-floor rows of joined metal seating facing a raised stage, noisy acoustics, the space echoing with scuffing feet, banging seats, talk and laughter. The facilitators are there, some of them standing around the hall, some scattered across the front row seats, among a number of the year 11 students who have arrived early. Graham has been mingling with the group of students in the front rows, engaging them in conversation, asking them questions about themselves. It's a cold morning and he's wearing a heavy winter coat – I've come to recognise this as a 'prop' in the latest variation of his introduction.

Once most of the students are in the hall and seated the school coordinator – a 30-something male teacher – raises his voice above the noise to attract their attention. 'You are about to be educated in what is probably one of the most important moral subjects, journeys that any area of high school can teach. I tell you from experience, as someone who knows, as a twelve year old, what it's like to drive a car into a tree.' There's some laughter at this, and the teacher is at pains to make his point: '… the tree remains where it is, the car (smashes) and you go flying.' Perhaps feeling like the point didn't really come across, he finishes with some emphasis: 'I want you to pay attention today, as the people conduct their seminar.'

There's extended applause from the students as Graham takes his place at the front of the stage. Acknowledging the welcome, he says, 'thank you indeed for giving us a clap, and thank you to the people' (nodding at some students in front of him) 'who came up the front here and introduced themselves to us.' He connects with the group by acknowledging his own nervousness. 'When coming to a group like this I've got to tell you, you actually get incredibly nervous. You don't know who I am, though I'm about to introduce myself; I don't know who you are. And I'm suddenly standing up here and I think: Urgh, what are you going to think?'

He indicates the Fit to Drive people around the hall, noting the 'group of people who are going to be working with you. We'll all raise our hands so we can show you how many of us there are. Round the room as well.' The students swivel in their seats to get a look at the facilitators, who are sheepishly raising their hands, as Graham continues: 'And we are here today, and this has already been said … to not say you're bad drivers, absolutely not … but we are here to tell you about how you are overrepresented in road crashes, and what you can do about it. So that's what we're going to do.

'First of all a little bit about me. I look as though I'm a … a transport inspector don't I?' Scattered laughter. Graham continues the joke: 'My wife always says to me, when we're travelling by public transport – and I usually do – Graham why are you wearing that coat? People think you're an inspector. When we sit on the tram or train everyone gets up and walks away.' More laughter. 'I'm not a transport inspector, but if you go beneath the coat you get a sense of who – or what – I might be.' Unbuttoning the coat to reveal his suit and tie, he confesses, 'I'm a former school principal.' Ruefully, he smiles and nods, acknowledging the reaction: 'Oh … I heard that groan!' Laughter. 'A former school principal, but it does show, and I am going to tell you about how my life was changed as a school principal and why I'm here today.' Before continuing he notes his connection with the area – he was born in the next suburb – and points out one of the facilitators who actually went to the school. His tone then changes, and his demeanour becomes serious.

'What I want to do is capture the moment though, when my life changed, and it changed as principal – why? I had been a principal for many years, I was a principal of a very large college down in Frankston – seventeen hundred and fifty students and a hundred and fifty staff, and I remember, that particular Friday …

'And in our school, we had a student by the name of Julie. Julie was in year 12, and with seventeen hundred and fifty students students, I believe every student knew Julie. She had been very, very prominent, because at that time there was a program called the Rock Eisteddfod.[1] *Not a lot of people know about the Rock Eisteddfod now, but it was big news in schools. Schools competed in the Rock Eisteddfod, and my school had actually won the state championship, and they had gone on to win a national championship, and Julie had figured prominently in that, so she had been on TV, and was known by everybody.*

'But, what happened was this. She came into what we called our common room, what you might call your VCE study area, and she came in, she walked in, and it was Friday, at the end of the day, and she just walked in and she went …' (Graham throws his keys down with a clatter on the stage behind him) '… with her car keys on the table, and across the way was her best friend, Ingrid, and she said to Ingrid … she'd had her licence for two weeks – and this was a time before 120 hours of experience … and she said "I've got my car here today, I'll drive you home." Her father had bought her a nearly new car, a Hyundai – he wanted her to be safe. So Julie said, "I'll drive you home."'

Graham's narration, dotted with asides, occasional repetitions and awkwardness, nevertheless flows with a studied, practised pace and intonation, timed for maximum impact. The pauses, shifts from loud to soft, the declamatory to intimate voice, add to the drama of the delivery and rhetorical impact. He uses gestures, body movement and position in the space to theatrical effect.

'And sitting across here was a boy – can anyone guess what this boy said?'

A young male student answers from the audience. I miss this, but Graham, thanking him and asking his name, picks up the cue: 'Absolutely what you'd expect a boy to say in those circumstances: "Can you drive me home too?" Julie said, "Yeah – I'll give you a lift." And the boy said, "Oh, by the way … I live in Hastings." Now, Hastings is a bit like living out at Mayfield, about that sort of distance, not just up the road. He said, "Look don't worry, let's go down to the station and I'll catch the train." So they head off, out the car park, past the gym and out on to the road, down the road to the station, and just as they got to the station they see the train to Hastings, going choof choof choof down the track. Now you're laughing because I say "choof choof."' (Though this is not why I'm laughing – a quick look around at the students confirms my guess at their interpretation – a row of boys are miming smoking weed. But the laughter is good-natured, and the students, whether or not they've picked up the unintended double-meaning, seem to be with the story, and accept Graham's image of the old steam train making its way out of the station.) 'If you see the train to Hastings', continues Graham, 'that's what it does – it goes choof choof choof, choof.' (more laughter) 'So out it went. And Julie said, "Look, I'll drive you – I said I'll drive you," so that's what they did, off to Hastings. And she dropped the boy off.'

Graham's voice drops very low; he steps back and leans against the stage behind him. The audience is quiet. 'I know what happened in that car. Julie and Ingrid were driving back and they were really pumped up, and they were talking about their netball match that they were going to play the next day. They had music on in the car, and they were really excited. They drew up, on an angle, at an intersection, and Julie, through inexperience, pushed out and along came a truck …'

The gasps and drawn-out groans from the audience fill the hall. Rather than a private intake of breath, this is a collective expression of shock. 'Julie was instantly killed. Ingrid was airlifted to hospital, and eventually recovered. I heard about it one hour later.' (Graham's body language: drawn in upon himself, looking down at his hands, held tightly to his body.) He says quietly, 'Julie's family have never recovered. They never will recover.

'I sat on the edge of the bed in Julie's bedroom with her Mum. We wept. And we looked around the room, looked at all of the pictures that were there, of her life, as it was till now. Gone.'

You can feel Graham re-living this moment, as his gestures, taking in different points around the hall, evoke the remembered images round Julie's room. He takes a brief moment to reflect. 'And I, from my perspective, I will forever remember the assembly that I held – it happened on the Friday, I held it on the

Monday. When I walked in to the assembly area, and it was like it is now – you could hear a pin drop. Everybody knew what I was going to say. Big school – we had three assemblies, I had to be at every one. And then, it got worse … we didn't think it could get any worse. Because in the space of eighteen months, seven young people, young drivers, were killed on the roads in our community. Seven of them. What happened out of that was a group of students came into my office. We talked with a group of staff, I met with a group of principals and we said, what can we do to change the circumstances so that this doesn't happen again? What do we do? And we set ourselves on a journey to find out: what's the best way, to actually involve young people to make sure it doesn't happen again?' His voice lightens here. 'It was an amazing time. In the first place we went to all of the experts – we were getting advice from everybody at that point in time. And you know, there were people who said this: What young people need is to be shocked. They need to be traumatised, they need to go into a morgue, they need to go into hospitals – see what actually happens.'

Graham moves down the aisle, into the audience space, as he's speaking. The tone is intimate, inviting the students to enter into the experience. 'Can you imagine, a community that can be more shocked, than a community that has already had seven deaths? This community was already traumatised, they didn't need to be shocked.' He moves back to the front of the hall. 'And what we read, and found out about the research, the research told us this, that shock tactics work about this much' (holds his hands about a foot apart). 'We go in there, we are shocked, we are traumatised' (he holds his hand to his chest) 'and then we say, quite predictably, as we should, whew, I hope that doesn't happen to me, or if it does, it will be my number coming up. So we know that shock tactics by themselves don't work.'

'And then there was the group, and I've gotta say, there's a lot of blokes my age, and they'd say … they'd come to –' (quietly asking a young student in the front row his name) '"Oscar," they'd say, "listen Oscar, what you need is to get more skills, you need to get out there and find out what driving's all about. I've been driving for years and, you just don't know what it's about." Have you heard people talking about that? "You need more skills," etc., etc., etc. There's a lot of truth behind that, but there's also a lot of information that says, if we give you an advanced driving course right at the start, then you will crash more often. Can you believe that? The actual evidence, the tests that have been done throughout the world tell us that you actually crash more often. So that wasn't the answer. The answer … was right here in the room.' Graham's voice again drops a register, and adopts a more intimate tone, at the same time emphasising each word: 'Absolutely right here in the room. Because the truth of it is, you have brought the road toll down.'

He leans back, placing his hands on the stage floor behind him.

'I'm going to tell you about the good old days. The good old days when I learnt to drive in Brixton, in 1973 – the dinosaur era!' (laughter). 'In 1973 there were a million and a half less people, two million less cars, and we killed a thousand and thirty-four people in one year, a third of them people my age.

"Good old days." Now the truth of it is, in that time, Victoria has become the world leader and we have brought the road toll down – to the totally unacceptable figure of just under three hundred, at the moment, a third of that young people, two virtually every weekend.' Graham is moving back and forth in front of the stage, as he states this. He holds up his fingers to indicate the number, emphasising the statistics with his gestures. 'But we have brought it down, and I'll give you a great example of how you've done it. You are far more responsible than I was about drink driving. My mates used to say: "I was too drunk to walk so I drove."' (Graham comically mimics the stupid drunken talk. Laughter.) 'It's unbelievable isn't it, but that's what my mates used to say. The reality is that you look after your mates better. So the truth of it is, what we're going to be doing today is to take you on a journey where you can discover how you can make yourselves safer. So we're not going to put you behind the wheel … And how many people have their Ls?' (puts his hand in the air, inviting students to raise their hands, notes the numbers) 'Lots – you're doing the right thing with your 120 hours. What we're going to do for everybody in the room, is actually capture for you how you can make yourselves safer,' (striding up to the stage, where the video equipment sits in readiness) 'and we're going to do it in this particular way.' (preoccupied with working the computer) 'We're going to show you a short film, and then we'll briefly discuss it.'

Outrage; horror; pity. This is a scene which perhaps would have piqued the interest of the great German playwright Bertolt Brecht. We can imagine Brecht in the back of the theatre, chomping with magnificent sensual pleasure on his cigar, wrapped in his old overcoat, worker's cap perched comfortably on his head, mind racing around the puzzles of representing complex social phenomena on the stage – to poke and prod his audience into thinking. We invoke Brecht because, as we will argue shortly, his theory of theatre reveals interesting things about dominant ideas concerning the nature and place of emotion, not only in the theatre, but also more broadly as a feature of human existence.

Watching the opening scenes of the Fit to Drive performance, we might think of Brecht, who in the 1930s articulated a new purpose for modern theatre: 'pedagogy'. Brecht's 'didactic theatre' was opposed to what he saw as the mere entertainment spectacles filling the theatres of his day. Fit to Drive as theatre could not be claimed to fit the criteria of art, but we would like to draw on Brecht's writings on theatre as a useful starting point for considering some of the key questions in this chapter. Brecht was concerned throughout his career with the reshaping of theatre as a space for the dramatisation, or dramatic working-through of the 'hugely complex' problems, or conditions, emerging out of modern life. These complexities, advocated Brecht, needed to be simplified, and presented on stage in a new dramatic form. They were to serve theatre's new purpose: pedagogy (Brecht 1963, pp. 226–227).

Brecht's ideas relate not only to the didactic role of theatre, but also reflect some of the key tensions surrounding discourses of 'emotion' and 'reason', and embodiment, that had dominated modern western thought up to the period in which he was writing. Ideas about 'emotion' are in turn intimately linked to questions about values and ethical conduct which, we argue, are central to the Fit to Drive project.

In Chapter 1 we explored the way Fit to Drive creates a *theatrical* space, in which the unusual spectacle of so many new faces ('cast'), the stage setting, students as audience, the performance of the presenter, the 'tone' of the presentation, all contribute to the impression of Fit to Drive as theatre. The novelty and interest of the event is matched by the dramatic quality of the theme for the morning – road crashes and their impact on young people. This chapter explores the ways that the components of the Fit to Drive presentation – the message (which in many respects resembles a theatre script), emotional engagement and values – are combined in the introductory whole group assembly and establish the setting for the learning activities to follow. The first segment is essentially about establishing road safety and young people as a problem. It aims to convince the audience members of the critical importance of taking the issue seriously, and being motivated to modify their behaviour based on the knowledge they will gain as a result of the morning's workshop.

The chapter will focus on two factors that are integral to the way road safety is presented as a problem. First, the way Fit to Drive emphasises and engages emotions using oral stories, rhetorical strategies and through short films. Engagement with the emotions is central to young people connecting with the issue and messages, and is, we will argue, integral to the reasoning process that the workshop aims to stimulate. The first emotional connection made with the students in Fit to Drive occurs in the theatrical space of the prologue – the presenter's monologue in which he or she tells the affecting story of a young person who lost their life so suddenly on an unforgiving road. The themes of sadness, regret, loss and anger established here are woven throughout the workshop (though, perhaps paradoxically, students are also surprised to find themselves evaluating and remembering the workshop as 'fun' and 'enjoyable').

The second, related factor is the moral dimension, the engagement with values. The presentation in this section is essentially an attempt to engage the student audience in a sense of shared values around the value of human life, the waste of young lives, and, importantly, questions of personal responsibility and self-control. We will draw on and use the idea of 'moral emotions' exemplified in the work of Antonio Damasio (1999, 2005), Jack Katz (1999), Mary Midgley (1994, 2001, 2003), Martha Nussbaum (2001a, 2001b) and Mark Johnson (1987, 2007) to discuss how Fit to Drive engages emotions as part of a transformative project.

We discuss these questions later in this chapter, but first we will explore the pedagogical, or 'didactic' core of the program.

Health education, youth work and values

If Fit to Drive is theatre, its purpose is clearly didactic. The teaching methods employed in the program, which are essentially engaging, interactive and participatory, do not preclude, and indeed support, the didactic nature of its purpose. How would we best characterise the pedagogical intent of the Fit to Drive program, and the educational philosophy that informs it? A useful starting point, once again, is to look to the origins of the program, and unearth the various influences that worked to mould it into its distinctive character. This excavation reveals the fundamental values that are at the heart of Fit to Drive, both as a force that shaped the program, and as the core of the program's 'message'.

The original design of the Fit to Drive program arose out of the combined experience of the developers in our respective (complementary) areas of professional practice. The educational philosophy informed by Graham's practice as teacher, published curriculum developer and school principal. Bern, following her youth work degree, had trained as a secondary teacher, but had returned after a year in the classroom to youth work. In addition to her community-based youth work practice, she had conducted group discussion programs for newly licensed young drivers in the pilot program, 'Reducing the Toll'. Kerry's contribution was shaped by her background in health promotion and youth work practice. VicRoads and the TAC contributed expertise and advice in relation to the specific road safety messages and 'do's and don'ts' of road safety education, later included in the Young Driver Resource (VicRoads 2005). These included, for example, the promotion of 120 hours practice as a learner driver – this was prior to legislation stipulating this as part of the graduated licensing policy, introduced in 2007 (Healy et al. 2012) and discouragement of certain practices such as shock tactics or off-road 'advanced driving skills' training. However, there was limited attention paid to the documentation, and systematic analysis and presentation of the theoretical foundations of the program, although in presentations, reports and training there was reference to some of the academic literature relating to current research that analysed 'best practice' in prevention and health promotion (Nation et al. 2003; Spruijt-Metz 1999).

The program was, in one sense, continuing a form of youth work into the school setting. This incorporated certain ideas about the nature of youth work as a distinct area of professional practice. Youth work was grounded in the building of relationships with young people (Smith 1988; Ingram and Harris 2001; Spence et al. 2006) and belief in the transformative nature of these relationships (for the young person and the worker). It also embraced practice based on advocacy, promotion of rights, and creation of opportunities for young people to flourish in creative partnerships (Patel 2010; Batsleer and Davies 2010). It is against this background that we now reflect on the values – and the place of values – in Fit to Drive.

The youth work practised in health promotion, whether in group programs, or general health service provision, is in sympathy with the practice of health education in its definition as an opportunity for people to explore, define, re-affirm or challenge their own values and beliefs, within an environment that involved connections with others. This is why so often – though certainly not solely – health education is conducted in group settings (Carmody 2009).

Health education literature commonly refers to the need for recipients of health information to assimilate (new) knowledge in relation to health issues in the context of the attitudes and beliefs that attend the issue. For instance, information about 'healthy eating' is understood, and made sense of, in the context of beliefs about, for example, the meaning of food, the exercise of control in relation to food as an indicator of moral worth and even social status, or the relationship between food choices and cultural identity (Pike and Kelly 2014; Pike and Colqhoun 2010; Probyn 2010).

A person's understanding and action in relation to any particular health issue will be built upon her or his established attitudes and beliefs about the issue itself (as in the case of food and healthy eating), as well as attitudes towards broader questions of self and of the self in the social setting. But how much of this understanding and conduct is rational and reflexively available to us? Pierre Bourdieu (1990) has written extensively about the sedimented nature of human practice-as-*habitus*. For Bourdieu *habitus* is suggestive of that set of established ways of thinking, feeling, and using our bodies as if the way we live is both the only and the natural way to live. Bourdieu (1990, p. 53) conceptualises *habitus* as the 'conditionings' associated with particular conditions of existence producing 'systems of durable, transposable dispositions which … generate and organize practices and representations'. Bourdieu (1990, p. 74) has stressed that so much of what we believe or claim to know, as well as so much of our behaviour, our bodily orientation in/to the world, is unconscious. It is through immersion in the myriad products, objects and practices of culture – verbal, material and social – that a person acquires, or grows into, *habitus*. Habitus is acquired in practice, in embodied actions, and practices are charged with 'a host of special meanings and values'. Bourdieu's conceptualisation of habitus has enabled writers to think about the way practices surrounding health-related behaviours are deeply embedded in dispositions reflecting 'value systems, behavioural norms, body perceptions' (Abel 2007, p. 43).

There is an extensive literature about the construction of the self as 'healthy citizen' (Lupton 1995; Ziguras 2004) and the various theories about the effects of class, culture and the social world on this form of citizen (Balbo 2007; Abel 2007). Common to the different accounts of health and the subject is the acknowledgement that individual behaviours are complexly embedded in attitudes and beliefs that are firmly located within the context of their social milieu. These beliefs are, in turn, grounded in the core values that have developed within the individual over a lifetime. An individual's values are at the foundation of action, their being in the world. In this sense a fundamental question for Fit to Drive is: How are we to change ways of feeling, thinking or doing that are palpably dangerous or harmful?

The question of values goes to the heart of debates about the nature of youth work practice and identity. Some writers have attempted to delineate a set of principles, attached to core values, which define the specific character and practice of youth work (Corney 2006). The identification of key values has been viewed as an indispensable part of the process of defining youth work. Judith Bessant's (2009, p. 438) discussion of virtue ethics and youth work practice has extended the enquiry by exploring the ethical frameworks at the foundation of practice, arguing that it is necessary to be able to articulate the 'social goods' that youth work promotes. Virtue ethics, with its focus on character, or 'virtues', its clear definition of 'social goods', and emphasis on the exercise of good judgement within a framework of these social goods, provides a 'better ethical guide for youth work practice'. It provides 'clear and helpful descriptions of social goods and the ways we may live a good life', with an emphasis on the role of character: 'The idea of "virtue" itself refers to good habits and dispositions to display character traits like courage, prudence, rationality or temperance'. This framework also provides a way of thinking about the transformative nature of youth work practice in that it proceeds from an understanding of young people as having agency – a capacity to change, grow and develop (skills, knowledge, attitudes and good judgement). This thinking stands in contrast with determinist views of young people as locked in their biology – whether hormonal or neurological – with limited agency.

Bessant (2009, pp. 432–434) highlights the importance accorded to education in the virtue ethics tradition: 'One strength of the virtue ethics tradition is its conviction that the virtues can be learnt and that good character is the product of a good education'. The tradition of virtue ethics 'warrants a degree of optimism about the value of education and training as the basis for developing good judgement', that is, to make good choices:

> to build character as a source of social transformation, its emphasis on our agential capacity to make choices, its interest in our capacity to think critically and act ethically, the connections it makes between the practice of virtues and social goods that define a good life individually or collectively.
>
> (Bessant 2009, p. 436)

This notion of ethics is firmly embedded in the very practical question of 'how we are to conduct ourselves in a rapidly changing and complexifying world?' (Grayling 2007, p. 187). This is an ethics securely rooted in 'human needs and values' and is concerned with the promotion of moral sensibility. Moral questions (in Grayling's sense) are concerned with 'the life of human beings in their social setting'; they arise from a 'felt need' – that is, they concern practical questions grounded in everyday life. The constantly changing landscape of contemporary life reinforces the urgency of employing an ethics that is capable of being a guide to moral conduct. Given the ongoing and everyday nature of moral choices, this is 'a task that requires reflection and continued negotiation'. Michel Foucault (1985, 1986) and Zygmunt Bauman

(2008) also take up these challenges, though from different directions and with different purposes. An important role of education in this context is the development of moral understanding, and knowledge of the self, in relation to questions of conduct in the world. An intrinsic part of this process involves an examination of personal values (see Jarvis 2006) and exposure to different viewpoints and ways of seeing the world.

Fit to Drive explicitly builds in engagement and teaching strategies that are about exploring values, building self-knowledge, and thinking about moral conduct – in relation to driving, but also by their very nature extended to broader applications of character virtues like prudence, rationality, compassion and the development of good judgement. In essence, the program contributes to, and is an extension of, the moral education of young people. The small group activities contribute to the development of self-knowledge, for example, by inviting students to think about their motivations in relation to choices and decisions, their values in relation to driving, and the implications of individual decisions and actions for others. Across the workshop the emphasis is on dialogue, and engagement with students is conducted, where possible, on the level of conversation: exploring and sharing beliefs and attitudes and experiences. The activities create space for the differing values and opinions within the group. The facilitator at the beginning of the 'Values' activity, in an endeavour to encourage open conversation, informs the group: '*There are no right or wrong answers.*' However, the intention is to provide a supportive environment where students' values and opinions may be challenged, and new views formed. The Fit to Drive message is explicit, as are the values that inform the program. These include appeals to maturity and responsibility, with the affirmation of young people as agents with the capacity to make choices, and to 'take ownership and responsibility for their own and their peers' safety'. The program's aims include fostering 'respect and pride in safe road use' (Spencer and Montero 2011, p. 3).

Affirmation of the value of human life and individual responsibility to others pervades the Fit to Drive message. The awareness of connection with others is present, for example, in the 'consequences' segment of the Monavale activity, in the stories, and in the films, where much of the power of the impact lies in the visible impacts on others. The personal (suffering, guilt, injury, death) is experienced on an individual level. But it is also accompanied by the strong sense of the social, interpersonal connections, and responsibility. These dimensions are reflected in the title of the peer education workshop that is part of the year 12 Fit to Drive program: 'Looking after your mates'. Students are asked to make, not just self-preserving decisions, but also choices about how they will act towards others, how they will comport themselves in relation to friends, community and the broader social body. Adopting moral behaviour – behaviour that goes against the peer or reference group – is an example of practising the virtue of courage. As educational theorist Peter Jarvis (2006, p. 49) notes, 'moral behaviour often demands confidence or courage'.

What is the relationship between values, moral choices and emotion? The role of emotion in developing values associated with the virtues and moral choices is a vexed question, and one of central importance to an analysis of the Fit to Drive program. Morality, though not specifically described in this language, is an essential concern of Fit to Drive, and is relevant to questions of emotion and reasoning. We have described how students are provoked to make, not just self-preserving decisions, but also choices about how they will act towards others, how they will comport themselves in relation to friends, community and the broader social body. Fit to Drive activities stimulate students to think about their values, specifically in relation to driving, but also in relation to their personal and social lives. As they consider choices and options, beliefs and opinions – that is, engage their reason – they also draw from the well-springs of their emotional selves.

Interlude: Brecht and the 'theatre of emotions'

What would Brecht have made of the emotionally charged introduction to the Fit to Drive workshop? Brecht was scathing of theatre that engendered a warm surrender to sentiment. In the poem 'Theatre of Emotions' (1976) he berates the sentimental dramatists whose sole interest is in staging plays that will pander to the sentimental tastes of lazy audiences. For Brecht, feelings are self-evidently 'inert', resembling lifeless, redundant, even parasitic, objects.

Brecht's instructions on how to engender the ideal theatre experience for an audience were all about fostering a 'critical attitude'. This was to be achieved by the content and form of the subject matter, the themes and problems of the drama, but also by the theatrical experience itself. Brecht's ideas about the creation of what he termed an 'alienation effect' were essentially about making the familiar 'strange'. For Brecht this meant creating the conditions under which the audience would be prepared to see things in a new light: not checking in one's brain in the cloakroom ('keep your overcoat on, your cigar in your mouth'). It was about illumination, figuratively and literally (keeping the house lights on). In short, it was about engaging *rationality*. Crucially, it was about avoiding a descent into the sentimentality and 'cheap emotion', which he saw in the popular theatre of his day.

Brecht's advocacy of a new kind of theatre that would seek to abandon cheap sentiment, and stimulate instead an analytical, critical orientation to the political and social themes and issues presented on the stage, emanated from his own political interests. This was an expression of his opposition to contemporary theatre which he saw as a crude 'masseur' of the bourgeoisie's self-satisfaction and as a means of bolstering their interests and stranglehold on art, as well as political and economic power.

We draw on Brecht's writings here because his interests were at the same time an expression of a deep and persistent ambivalence that has run through western thought about the role and value of feelings. This ambivalence has been expressed on the one hand as a concern with, and elevation of, an idea of Reason, and the Rational, that was at the heart of western philosophical and scientific thinking in modernity. A counterbalance to this dominance has been consistently evident in the writings of thinkers from Plato through to Hume, who offers a classically ambivalent account of feelings (Hume 2007), and may be seen in the (post)modern recovery of emotions as cognitively and ethically valuable.

The emotion Brecht speaks of is associated with an unthinking, passive response to stimuli, the opposite of critical thinking. The strands of this critique of emotion (or its even lowlier variant, sentiment) are to be traced to the rationalist tradition in modern western thought, a trajectory that privileged rationality, enshrined as Reason, over a notion of Emotion as a manifestation of the baser aspects of humanity.

The Age of Reason, or Enlightenment, has relegated emotions to the bottom drawer of human existence. Opposed to, and in struggle with this, are the 'higher faculties' of Reason and Rationality. The mind, with its 'machine-like' capacities for calculation, was venerated as the domain of Reason, and contrasted with the baser workings of emotions (Lupton 1998; Midgley 1994, 2003). Rationality, rational thinking, was work undertaken by cognitive processes in the mind, distinct from emotion (and the senses). It was the conduit to true knowledge. Truth is produced along the path of logical thought sequences.

The dichotomies established within modernity between reason and emotion (of which the mind/body, culture/nature, human/animal, male/female oppositions are also an expression) have had a profound impact on ideas about who we are as human beings. The idea of the human being who is composed of an 'emotional self' and a separate, 'reasoning' self is one that has dominated western thought and has formed a foundational truth in various fields of human studies and systems of practice. Drawing on older knowledge, and moral schemes imagining competing personal and cosmic forces (of, for instance, good and evil), ideas about human nature have been accompanied by assumptions of separate, warring aspects of the psyche, that wage a battle for ascendancy. Hume, for example, referred to a conflict between Passion and Reason, 'with Reason the Slave of the Passions' (Midgley 2003).

Emotions belonged to the realm of the corporeal, connected with the instincts, drives and the passions, and were associated with the negative view of the body in Christian orthodoxy. These were the aspects of being human that were equated with nature, the biological. As Lupton (1998, p. 3) argues: 'Because the emotions are viewed as embodied sensations, they are considered to be the antithesis of reason and rationality'. Emotion continued, within this tradition, to be associated with instinct, the body, the primitive, and was therefore in need of taming, regulation and mastery: 'From this perspective, the emotions are impediments to proper considered judgement and intellectual activity' (Lupton 1998, p. 3). For many socio-cultural theorists emotions were associated with the body, and therefore possibly tainted with social-Darwinist, biological determinist, perspectives on human experience (Lupton 1998, p. 2).

The view of the emotions as impeding a person's capacity to reason, and as an expression of the baser aspects of human existence, and the uninformed mind in particular, continued to be dominant throughout the nineteenth and much of the twentieth centuries. In one sense Brecht is an exemplar of that tradition of Marxist critical thinking that practises an austere 'critical rationality' that punctures illusion, false sentimentality and ideology, and portrays the audience of this 'theatre of emotions' as 'glassy-eyed', preferring to 'sit in the dark that hides them' (Brecht 1976). Brecht's expression of contempt for emotion – the 'theatre of emotion' – is at the same time part of a century-old tradition of radical critique of the German middle classes, who were perceived as smug, comfortable and reactionary. This was a critique that associated emotion – 'sentiment' – with all that was intellectually lazy, complacent and politically dangerous in human society. Brecht, in keeping with this tradition, rejects the blatantly sentimental, which he sees as a shoddy attempt to entertain and titillate self-righteous audiences, whom he likens to voyeurs, wallowing in manufactured emotions that are murky, hypocritical and self-satisfied.

Is Fit to Drive an example of theatre of emotion? An appeal to emotion, even sentimentality, through the stories of horrific crashes, in order to provoke a response in young people? In sensationalising and sentimentalising the 'tragic' is it merely a version of the tactics the media are often accused of?

If we take the key messages of Fit to Drive as relating to questions of moral conduct we arrive at the nub of one of the core disputes concerning rationality and emotion. Philosopher Mary Midgley (2003, p. 5), exploring the arguments about the rational and emotional aspects of human experience, examines these debates in the context of moral philosophy. She describes the way British moral philosophy 'from the eighteenth century on has occupied itself with a dispute about whether morality is a matter of reason or feeling', a position that ignores, as Midgley observes, 'the obvious fact that it's both'. Moral philosophy was perhaps not capable of imagining a 'both' when it came to questions of the rational and emotional.

This view of emotion hasn't gone unchallenged: 'Is emotion a sack of potatoes, so much the pound, to be measured out? Am I a machine? I shall be told I can use up my emotions by using them, next' (Forster 1987, p. 241). In his novel *A Passage to India* E. M. Forster has his Indian character, Aziz, make this speech in response to his English friend Fielding. The speech reflects the puzzlement and exasperation of the character to the perceived coldness of even the most sympathetic of the English colonialists. This is a revealing moment in the novel. Forster depicts an ultimately unbridgeable gulf between the English and Indians that is made manifest in their different ideas about, more accurately, their different feelings about, emotion. The response is made even more significant by the fact that Aziz is a doctor, trained in western medical science, and embracing of 'modern thinking'. It is telling that Forster's description of Aziz's retreat from a connection with European sensibilities towards the end of the novel is associated with his return to emotions as the guiding force for his thinking, and conduct: 'Aziz had no sense of evidence. The sequence of his emotions decided his beliefs' (Forster 1987, p. 260).

Rediscovering emotions

Counter-discourses that valued the emotions as an important aspect of human being existed alongside the view of emotion as impediment to rational thought, both in academic literature and systems of knowledge/practice, as well as lay understandings. In certain social circles in the eighteenth century, for instance, the cult of the sentimental was a direct reaction to the perceived coldness and calculation of the Enlightenment *philosophes* (Leventhal 1994).

The neglect of, and disdain for, the emotions was also challenged by Romantic philosophy and the arts, where the emotions were seen as the expression of an essential aspect of our 'selves' – spontaneous, natural, untainted by culture and society, 'authentic'. For the Romantics, emotions were the 'well-springs for human action' (Lupton 1998, p. 81). These ideas were further explored in later Romantic and existentialist philosophy.

The past few decades have witnessed further challenges to the dismissal of the emotions in various fields of human studies. Midgley (2003, pp. 100–102) argues for an understanding of the emotions that places them at the core of the reasoning process and challenges those who separate, and oppose, rationality and emotion. Referring to the 'logic of the emotions' she declares: 'All dramatizations which set Reason as one participant against other aspects of the personality are confused'. Midgley (2003, p. 6) is arguing for the unity of emotion and rationality from the perspective of moral philosophy, observing that:

> Morality, like every other aspect of human activity, has both its emotional and its intellectual side, and connection between them can't be just an external one, like that between stones brought together for a building. It is an organic one, like that between the shape and size of an insect.

Similarly, Martha Nussbaum (2001b, p. xxvii) has argued for rejection of the 'reason/emotion dichotomy' and for the recognition of the central place of emotions in reason and rationality and their role in 'informing us about matters of ethical significance'. From the perspective of recent developments in social theory, 'emotional experience is considered to be an essential and insightful conduit to knowledge' (Lupton 1998, p. 3). Emotional responses are viewed as 'important sources of human values and ethics and as a proper basis for political action' (ibid.). Lupton (1998, p. 4) is mainly referring here to the emotional engagement of the academic, and the 'emotional under-pinnings of academic research, scholarship and teaching', but the insight has wider application.

The view that emotion is intricately involved in the development of learning and the process of reasoning, has also found support in fields of psychology and, more recently, in developments in neuropsychology. The neuroscientist Antonio Damasio (2005, p. xi), grounding his claims in neuro-biological studies, proposes that emotion is an intrinsic part of the reasoning process, and notes that emotion is 'in the loop of reasoning, and … could assist the reasoning process rather than necessarily disturb it, as was commonly assumed'. Damasio (2005, p. xii) argues that: 'When emotion is entirely left out of the reasoning picture, as happens in certain neurological conditions, reason turns out to be even more flawed than when emotion plays bad tricks on our decisions'. Damasio (2005, p. xiii) rejects the emotional brain/reasoning brain paradigm: 'Clearly I never wished to set emotion against reason, but rather see emotion as at least assisting reason and at best holding a dialogue with it'. Rather than seeing emotion as opposed to cognition, he affirms emotion 'as delivering cognitive information, directly and via feelings'.

Mark Johnson (2007), in his study of the bodily basis of human meaning making, extends the investigation into the role of feelings and emotions in human knowing. Rejecting models of knowing and meaning making that assume the existence of a disembodied mind, Johnson (2007, p. x) draws from pragmatist philosophical traditions (James 1890/1950; Dewey 1997), phenomenology (Merleau-Ponty 2008; Gendlin 1962, 1995) and 'second-wave' cognitive sciences, to explore the 'deep, visceral origins of meaning'. Johnson (2007, p. 9) argues that there 'is no cognition without emotion, even though we are often unaware of the emotional aspects of our thinking'. Johnson further emphasises the 'central role of emotion in how we make sense of our world'. Building on the pragmatists' conceptualisation of body/mind as a continuity, Johnson (2007, p. xi) observes that meaning 'is not just a matter of concepts and propositions'. Rather, meaning making also 'reaches down into the images, sensorimotor schemas, feelings, qualities and emotions that constitute our meaningful encounter with our world'.

This insight has implications for human learning. Existentialism, according to educational theorist Peter Jarvis (2006, p. 4), teaches us to understand learning as an 'essential element of Being'. 'Learning … lies at the heart of our humanity – it is a driving force in human existence'. Theories of human learning have investigated and affirmed the central place of our emotions: we learn 'from and through our feelings'. 'At the heart of all learning is not merely what is learned, but what the learner is becoming (learning) as a result of doing and thinking – and feeling' (Jarvis 2006, p. 6). Learning theorists recognise both the obstructive impact of emotions on learning (excessive anxiety) as well as the inextricable relationship of emotions to the process of learning. In Jarvis' model of human learning, learning is identified as occurring when a person has experienced a disjuncture from a previously taken-for-granted world, and this experience is necessarily accompanied by a range of emotions – 'we feel unease, disharmony, and may lack self-confidence and so on'. Jarvis (2006, p. 19) notes that the process of resolving the disharmony through learning involves other emotions. 'Emotions can have a considerable effect on the way we think, on motivation and on beliefs, attitudes and values'. Emphasising the nature of learning as a transformative experience, Jarvis (2006, p. 21) describes this as a process whereby we transform the content of our experiences (sensations) 'by thought, action or emotion, or by any combination of them'.

We have argued that Fit to Drive works – sometimes comfortably, sometimes with more ambiguity – within this tradition that recognises the place of emotion in meaning making and, by extension, learning. Sometimes, however, emotion seems to be set against reason, re-emerging as the old dichotomy, in ways that were emphatically brought home when visiting a workshop after a period of absence.

Interlude: 'Fridays with Graham', November 2009. Talking about feelings, behaviours, consequences

I'm travelling back from Castlereagh Secondary College with Graham, where I have been observing a workshop with around a hundred year 11 students. It's our first chance to catch up and chat for a while and, as always, our conversation meanders around several topics before we settle down to dissecting the day's program. It's been a while since I've observed a workshop, and I'm curious about some innovations that have been introduced.

I sat in with 'Briony', an experienced facilitator, for the second small group workshop, and was curious about changes to the last activity. This activity has the group working with a problem solving scenario and devising solutions, with phrases they can use to assertively put themselves out of danger. One scenario involves the young person as passenger in a car with a friend, who is driving erratically and too fast, because they have had a fight and the friend is angry. The idea is to illustrate how the emotions (particularly anger, distress, etc.) can prevent the exercise of rational responses to situations, and can lead to rash, in this case dangerous, behaviour. The students come up with some strategies to make the driver slow down and role-play the scenario, practising the phrases they would say. The facilitator writes them on the whiteboard, and discusses with the group the impact of the emotions on thinking and decision making. On this occasion Briony had drawn a circle, with a wavy line across the middle. In the top half she wrote 'Emotion' and the bottom half 'Rational'. 'What happens', she asked the group, 'when the emotions are high – you're angry or upset?' The students got it: the emotional bit takes up more of the circle, and the rational bit shrinks. The point is, explained Briony, 'We want to bring down the emotions, and raise the rational thinking'.

The schema was familiar. This way of framing the relationship between the emotions and the 'thinking self' was adapted by Bern from Bolton's 'People Skills' (Bolton 1986) and introduced to facilitator training. It is a way to think about being clear-headed, making good decisions, and the impact of heightened emotions on rational thinking. I hadn't realised it had been introduced as a tool for the facilitators to use, as a way of summarising the learning in the workshop. What did I think of that? The question was unsettling me, for some reason.

The activity graphically illustrates the enduring positioning of emotion in opposition to rationality. The rational/emotional circle innovation further accentuates the view that emotions are fundamentally problematic, even dangerous. The implications for young people are multiplied: dominant discourses about young people position them as irrational, subject to rash impulses, and as engaging in reckless, even dangerous, behaviour. They are seen to be at the mercy of biological forces, whether hormonal or neurological. Popular and expert discourses commonly describe them as hyper-emotional, with 'emotion' clearly laden with layers of negative associations. In young driver discourses the excessive emotionality of young people is an underlying theme that links to common explanations of their likelihood of being involved in a crash.

These perceptions of young people lead to the conclusion that, from the educator's (adult) perspective, emotion is a perilous genie to conjure with. Like the magic summoned by the Sorcerer's Apprentice, it can be a handy tool, but dangerous and prone to get out of control. Various discourses of emotion are discernible in the responses to, and management of, young people's reactions to the sudden death of friends and peers. Mourning rituals attending the sudden death of young people (particularly road trauma and suicide) are closely managed in school and institutional contexts (and youth work settings), to prevent expression of excessive and 'inappropriate' emotion. Yet expression of emotion (albeit carefully managed and directed) is seen as appropriate and 'healthy'. These parallel responses reflect the view of emotions, on the one hand, as an integral aspect of human existence, and on the other, as something that constantly threatens to tip us over into dark territory, associated with loss of control, failure of reason, and subjugation to powerful forces outside our true (rational) selves.

As a consequence, professionals and authorities are often careful of 'stirring up' emotion (there are echoes of wariness of mass hysteria here as well). In Fit to Drive there is a sensitivity to the emotional reaction of the students to the films, stories and discussion encountered during the workshop. Care is taken to support and care for students who might become emotional and schools are consulted beforehand to check whether there have been any incidents that would cause students to be exceptionally sensitive (for example a recent crash affecting students, or staff, in the school). Graham and I have been talking about the extra measures that were taken to prepare for a recent workshop at a school on the outer northern fringes of Melbourne, where emotion was running high following a triple road fatality in the area involving former students.

As a learning tool the rational/emotional circle is a potentially effective visual hook and memory aid. However, given that Fit to Drive draws on certain emotions to engage the students in thinking about moral decisions, are these positions in tension? Are there 'good emotions' and 'bad emotions'? Or are emotions neutral but nevertheless need to be 'managed'? When Briony continues to work with the scenario, getting students to suggest phrases for asserting their right to be safe in the car, she circles words that correspond to 'feelings', behaviours' and 'consequences', to which she allocates the abbreviation 'FBC'. For example: 'I feel unsafe (F) when I'm afraid.' (Other consequences could be: 'we'll get pulled over by police', 'lose your licence', and so on.) This time the emotions are positive. They help to identify when a situation isn't 'right', isn't safe. Emotions are mobilised to identify the unsafe situation, and are used to convince the driver to respond to the passenger's requests.

Fit to Drive's orientation to the emotional/rational construct is at once a product of the dichotomous relationship that is part of a philosophical inheritance. At the same time it is a pragmatic understanding and use of the concepts to achieve specific results. For instance, the everyday uses of dualistic juxtapositions of rational/emotional, such as in the Scenario exercise, may be a useful way of thinking about personal conduct, and negotiating the social world. It recognises that for many, emotion, in the form of anger or anxiety, may act as an impediment to clear thinking. As Jarvis (2006, pp. 108–109) notes, in relation to the limitations of Golemans' analysis of the 'rational/emotional mind', Goleman's studies are popular, perhaps for the very reason that they 'make sense within the world of work that he discusses ... Since his suggestions are practical – they work'.

Health promotion and emotion as 'embodied sociality'

Road crashes, for most people, are part of the background noise of our culture. Evening news programs report on the dramatic details of road crashes on an almost daily basis. We become accustomed to seeing the images of car wrecks, overturned trucks and smashed motorbikes flash across our screens, accompanied by the grim commentary of the newsreaders, interviews with weary emergency service workers, visuals of court cases and traumatised, grieving relatives. Viewing these images we may momentarily experience sympathetic sorrow, outrage, hopelessness, and then move on. Emotions such as these are not normally sustained for long when removed from our immediate sphere of affect.

In the telling of the various Fit to Drive stories, in the viewing of the films, similar emotions will be evoked. Why should we expect the impact to be any less ephemeral than that of a nightly news program? Shouldn't the impression made by such events be just as fleeting? Yet feedback from the students at the end of the workshop tells us that they have been affected by the stories, and their emotional impact, and six months after the workshop, groups of students report changing their attitudes (and behaviours) on the basis of the workshop experience.

Emotions are not just an essential part of our 'selfhood', but are quintessentially social in nature. The expression of human emotion – the forms it takes, the reverberations of emotional excess on social groups and communities, the desirability of finding means to regulate emotional expression – has interested and concerned people across diverse cultures and historical epochs. Some studies of human emotions claim that we are able to identify commonalities of emotional expression across human cultural and social groups (Katz 1999). However, the way we experience, interpret and express emotion is to a large degree culturally and socially dependent. Much of the renewed interest in the emotions as 'phenomena that are shaped, experienced and interpreted through social and cultural processes' (Lupton 1998, p. 2) has come out of the field of sociology of the body, with its interest in the body as a socially constructed and regulated entity. 'Like the body itself, emotional states serve to bring together nature and culture in a seamless intermingling in which it is difficult to argue where one ends and the other begins' (Katz 1999, p. 3). Some have turned their attention to the place of emotion in social understandings of the self and the role of social relations in generating emotion. 'The self comes into being and is continually formed and reformed by virtue of its location in a social milieu' (Lyon 2009, p. 73). Buytendijk (1973) refers to 'emotional modes of being' to suggest 'the way in which relationships or aspects of social structure are experienced by individuals both cognitively and bodily'. As medical anthropologist Margaret Lyon (2009, p. 71) remarks, 'emotion provides the link between the body and the social world'. Lyon (2009, p. 69), declaring that 'emotion is at the foundation of human society', draws the link between emotion (as an inextricable part of the rational, reasoning process) and the social nature of human beings.

The human (and higher primate) affective capacity is both demonstrated in, and crucial to, the formation of strong relational/affective bonds, bonds, which undergird social life and thus, ultimately, are an important aspect of the fabric of society. Emotion is equally as important as, and inextricably linked to, the capacity for so-called logical or rational functions, and it is also implicated in instrumental action.

Citing the work of Collins (1984) on human emotion, which 'goes beyond a focus on the individual and considers the importance of feelings in coalitions, e.g. feelings of membership', Lyon (2009, p. 71) notes the importance of 'emotional group identification' which 'for Collins is accomplished through sets of what he terms "interaction ritual chains"'. The relationship between emotion and social relations or social existence poses interesting questions for the way programs such as Fit to Drive are experienced by their participants.

The tensions between understandings of reason and emotion play out in interesting ways in Fit to Drive. At first blush it would seem that the weight of the 'facts' of road safety on their own should lead young people to reason that the problem is one that demands serious attention, and an active response. The problem should be evident from a 'logical' reasoning process. Graham's workshop introduction is peppered with statements that appeal to facts and evidence: 'The research told us …', 'actual evidence shows …', 'tests that have been done throughout the world …', 'the fact is …' He quotes statistics to emphasise his point and lend weight to his argument. The case has been established for safe driving through rational argument and empirical evidence. Academic studies of the problem of young drivers have logically demonstrated, via statistical evidence, the characteristics of crashes and young people as the safest (learner drivers), or 'least safe' (novice drivers) population group. This information has been augmented by psychological studies and psychosocial analysis of young drivers. The full weight of scientific argument sits behind the Fit to Drive message. We can therefore engage our rationality in order to make 'safe choices', to exercise decision making. The 'factual evidence' plays an interesting additional role. In the wake of the emotional buffeting of the introductory story, the 'solid reality' of 'facts and stats' provides a metaphorical anchor point. It is a way of reclaiming certainty, and therefore control, when confronted with the unsettling effects of the overtly emotional dimensions of the subject. In so many respects it is this logical structure that gives shape to so many interventions and health promotion programs for young people, particularly in school contexts.

Also present in the discourses of Fit to Drive is the idea of emotion as impediment to right thinking and action, as dangerous, a thing to be struggled with, and controlled. This understanding of emotion reflects a commonly held understanding that people employ in their everyday lives (Lupton 1998, p. 69). This view is exemplified in the rational/emotional model used in the workshop where the aim is to 'bring down the emotional component'. Emotion is a force to be 'managed', controlled, in a rational/emotional battle. However, it is evident that emotion is also present and embraced as a positive influence. The emotional appeal is an integral part of the content of the program as well as a *technique* of engagement. This sits comfortably with studies of human knowledge, moral reasoning and learning that show us that these faculties are intricately intertwined with our emotions. Emotion is an integral component of the reasoning/cognitive process, whether or not the object of our reasoning is overtly 'emotional' in content. When the subject is as emotionally charged as young people and road trauma, the impact and expression of that emotion in the group setting may be viewed as something that requires monitoring and management.

In the Fit to Drive workshop the problem of young people and road safety is established for its audience by openly appealing to the emotional aspects of road trauma. Young people are invited to feel, and to think (and act) (Midgley 2003). It is recognised that they need to be emotionally engaged. Young people need to connect (identify) with the situation through stories and shared experience. It is, of course, also the case that the developers of the program are operating within the same condition: they wouldn't be able to conceive or design the enterprise outside of the emotional dimension, irrespective of their 'ideas' or communicated views about this. Just as we, as researchers, are both consciously and unconsciously affected by the emotional aspects of the subject.

What is the nature of the emotion that is present, expressed, felt – 'manufactured' or spontaneous – in the Fit to Drive workshop? How to analyse it, in the light of the complex and shifting meanings and attributes, the weight it carries, the neglect it has been subject to? In Fit to Drive 'emotion' reflects and carries the multiple meanings that have attached to the embodied experience, as well as the word itself. Emotion is part of what it is to be human, a conduit for understanding, and, therefore, intimately connected with morality and ethical conduct. It is socially engendered and experienced, the site where 'private feelings and public moralities' are brought together (Scheper-Hughes and Lock 1987). It is marked by some level of discomfort and concern that exists in relation to emotional content of public discourse and public display of emotion.

The affirmation of the importance of teaching young people strategies for reasoning and rational decision making has political significance as well. Understandings of young people as being ruled by their emotions, lacking capacity for rational thought and decision making, have no currency in the Fit to Drive program (Carr-Gregg 2007). The program adopts approaches based on the ideas of transformative education that affirm young people's capacity to learn – and the imperative to teach them – personal and interpersonal skills. Skills such as decision making, problem solving, negotiation, conflict management, communication, and conduct of relationships are as integral to the program as the facts and messages. Rationality, in the framework of virtue ethics, is one of the 'virtues' that can be taught.

Many of the limits and possibilities, the challenges and opportunities that emerge in engaging emotions, exploring values, mobilising rationality in Fit to Drive, and in health promotion with young people, will be taken up in different ways in the following chapter.

Note

1 A health promotion program in Australian schools that encouraged young people to participate in choreography, musical competition, to be drug-free, to be '100% be your best!'

4 'Do, then talk'

Young people, group work and the making of meaning

Does her body think?

Richard Flanagan, in his novel *Wanting*, has placed Lady Jane Franklin, wife of the colonial governor, on a beach in remote Flinders Island, off Van Diemen's Land in the mid-nineteenth century. At the ends of the earth, both physically and figuratively. She is accompanying her husband, Sir John Franklin, on his vice-regal inspection of the recently established 'settlement', site of the colonialist project to transport the Aboriginal people from Tasmania to be 'civilised and Christianised'. Flanagan describes Lady Jane's impressions of landing at a beach crowded with indigenous people expressing joyful, animated greeting. The uninhibited physical expression of their welcome presents a contrast to the reserved formality of the English party (Flanagan 2008, p. 49).

The meeting on the beach is a powerful symbolic moment in Flanagan's novel, one that echoes in historical accounts and literary representations of early indigenous–European encounters in Australia. Among the early records of sailors from the First Fleet are descriptions of all-too-brief moments in this history when traditional owners and invaders were able to experience a spontaneous moment of shared human being. Exchanging gifts, sharing a visual joke, or 'dancing with strangers' (Clendinnen 2005). The memories of those fleeting moments of shared experience, already tinged with consciousness of the stranger as 'Other', soon became lost in the history of European occupation of the country, bolstered by the technology of a culture that was confident of its own superior 'civilised' status.

It is as representatives of this superior culture that the governor's party benevolently observes the exuberant display on the beach, which had been at least partly orchestrated by the settlement's Protector of Aborigines, and staged as a spectacle for the visitors. Lady Jane is drawn to the sight of a young girl in the children's corroborree; eye-catching, not just because of the arresting image of the little black child with her beautiful necklace and cloak of white kangaroo skin. Rather, her attention is captured by something ineffable in the child's manner, her presence.

The child is Mathinna, who becomes a symbol and an object of Lady Jane's 'wanting' – her desires, the currents and stirrings of her body and psyche. Flanagan's novel takes up the story of the historical Mathinna, born on Flinders Island to parents whose first child had been kidnapped and held hostage as a means of forcing her father (an Aboriginal clan leader) to cede to the Aboriginal protector's demands to move to Flinders Island. Mathinna is adopted by Lady Jane and Sir John. She is then 'assimilated' into the family's privileged life in colonial Hobart, to later be abandoned on the couple's return to England.

Flanagan's novel is, among other things, about desire, wanting: the wanting that 'is a manifestation of the whole of life', to quote Dostoevsky's *Notes from Underground* that provides the epigraph at the beginning of the novel (Flanagan 2008). It is about the struggle to contain and control the passion through reason; and the price that is paid for that struggle. In the novel that struggle is played out against and within the war of extermination that was being perpetrated on the indigenous peoples of Tasmania. The problem of the body was central to that project. Control, regulation, containment, annihilation of bodies. Lady Jane is troubled by her own body. She is haunted by her body's failures, disgusted by her husband's body. For her, his very features, his flesh, the noises his body emits, are a grotesque reminder of our animal nature (Flanagan 2008, p. 55). She is unsettled by the currents and tides of her body, the unwelcome emotions that are visited on her, the sensation of 'falling' into deeply buried feelings. The sight of the young Aboriginal girl, Mathinna, dancing in the children's corroborree, following rhythms and knowledge of the world unknown to the observer, stirs a dormant bodily echo in the woman. Her own body responds: a sensation of release, opening the space for an unfamiliar emotion.

Dance occupies a liminal space here: somewhere between 'nature' and 'culture'. A conundrum for the European sensibility. A potentially uncomfortable reminder of the pleasures, the realities of the body, easily interpreted as a primitive expression of bodily passions. As Jane Austen's Mr Darcy sniffs: 'Every savage can dance' (Austen 1996, p. 24). The brief scene that follows the dance, rich in symbolic meaning, plays out in a swirl of Lady Jane's memories (miscarriages, silenced grief), witty, urbane allusions to the classical origins of the girl's European name (Leda) and the magnetic fascination of the child's dance on the beach. Uncharacteristically, Lady Jane is drawn to touch the child on the arm as she passes, a gesture that is unsettling for both.

Lady Jane recognises the significance of her experience. She deals with the disturbance this encounter has roused within in her by embarking energetically on the interrupted tour of the settlement, setting a gruelling pace for the rest of her party, her mind preoccupied with the thoughts and feelings following her encounter with Mathinna. Reflecting on the child's dancing, her movement, her body – so expressive, it seems to Lady Jane, of the child's experiences, emotions, the grief and loss so recently encountered – Lady Jane hesitates to express the inconceivable, but the question, for her, is compelling: can her body be said to *think*?

Embodied meaning making

In the Fit to Drive workshops there have been many moments where the physical, embodied, quality of the experience is particularly accented. 'Close your eyes', instructs Angela at the beginning of the MFB presentation. A hush descends on the auditorium as the students shut their eyes. Eyes closed, the young people draw on different senses, are opened to different sensations, as they follow the story.

At training, Bern takes the facilitators through one of the workshop activities so they can experience it as the young people do. As she finishes with the closing line she pauses, and asks the group to 'step to the side, put your facilitator hat on', to begin the 'how-to' of facilitating the activity. The physical movement signals the 'stepping into' the consciousness of becoming a facilitator.

On another occasion, over morning tea during a break in the workshop, a young woman is talking to Grant about her feelings after participating, as a volunteer, in a re-creation of the overcrowded car that features in the Monavale crash case study.[1] To set the scene, Grant had enlisted eight students, to their amusement, and the delight of the audience, to squash into the simulated 'car', just as the young partygoers had on the night of the fatal crash. The students weren't required to act out the trauma, just the chaos that reigned in the car. Amid the hilarity, Grant had simply pointed out the overcrowding, the distractions and the dangerous conditions that were accumulating in the vehicle. He had thanked the students and allowed them to return to their seats in the audience before describing the crash that occurred just a kilometre down the road from the party, and showing the short film about the crash and its consequences.

Later, in the break, the young woman is describing the impact of sitting in that 'car' (six moulded plastic chairs) and later learning of the young people's fate. It had been a profound feeling, she commented. She had felt a palpable connection with the young people's experience. She 'really understood it'. For the audience there is an imaginative leap involved in picturing, in empathising with the young people (as a foundation for critical reflection on their actions and decisions leading to their plight). For the young woman seated in the 'car', squashed in with the other girls, there was a different quality to this awareness. For her there was a direct link between her bodily experience and her understanding, her meaning making.

For Les Todres (2007, p. 2) the 'lived body grounds understanding by intimately participating in a world that can show new horizons and meanings. It is this participative and aesthetic dimension that the lived body gives to understanding.' For Todres (2007, p. 12) this aesthetic dimension extends to the very marrow of our being. We 'go through an experience' by means of our senses, which 'penetrate the fluid of our bodies' and thus enter into a new relationship with the world: 'a particular form of the world finds a home through our accommodating stance'. Of course, the students sitting down in the audience in the large group session are also constructing meaning and developing understanding within the flow of their experiencing – experiencing that is of a fundamentally embodied nature. But this particular young woman's experience is a particularly powerful illustration of this quality of meaning making as embodied process.

Lady Jane is intrigued by the strange notion: her body thinks. Her manner of framing the problem is characteristic of western, Cartesian, thinking about the mind – ideas that shaped, and continue to shape, modern scientific, western thinking. The mind/brain *thinks*, the body constitutes an uncomfortable, but necessary *other*. It is a machine of moving parts that responds to stimuli. Passions are an acceptable, even desirable element, if properly controlled and managed. Though sometimes, it would seem, the stimuli would need to be powerful indeed to move the machine to passion. Lady Jane, who thinks of her husband's body as having the approximate intelligence of a pumpkin (Flanagan 2008, p. 53), senses nevertheless that even this pumpkin-body harbours the germ – or embers – of passion, of spirit, waiting to be kindled.

Flanagan is plausibly reproducing, in Lady Jane Franklin, the assumptions of the era. He is at one level drawing on a tradition that perceives a fundamental dissonance between European (Enlightenment) relationships to the body, and the unconscious, integrated bodily awareness of indigenous peoples encountered by European colonists. The twentieth-century cognitive scientists who followed a century after the period in which the novel was set, favouring the computer metaphor of the mind, transfigured the idea of mind as machine into a view of consciousness, and of thinking, as an outcome of computational processes in the brain. The brain, in turn, was a passive receptor of 'input'. To say that the body *thinks* is to upend the established order, but Lady Jane's insight anticipates Merleau–Ponty's (2008) approach to cognition and consciousness that recognised thinking as beginning with, and within, the felt experience of the body. It is only recently that this approach has received sympathetic attention from 'phenomenology-friendly neuro-science' (Ellis 2006), or what Johnson calls 'second-wave cognitive science' (Johnson 2007). There is a growing theoretical recognition of the bodily basis of cognitive thinking, and the phenomenological foundations of human meaning making (Damasio 1999; Gendlin 1991; Noe 2009).

We are accustomed to the idea that the body reacts to 'external' experiences. External stimuli may be unconsciously 'internalised', and manifest at some point as bodily responses, reactions and changes. However, until recently it has been a radical idea to propose that bodily sensations and feelings form an essential ground for thinking, that there is a 'felt quality' (Johnson 2007, p. 94) to logical relations prior, and necessary to, thinking:

> The idea that thinking is embodied is not the relatively obvious claim that in order to think, one needs a body and a brain. Instead, it entails that the nature of our embodiment shapes both what and how we think, and that every thought implicates a certain bodily awareness.
>
> (Ibid.)

From the acceptance of the bodily basis of cognitive processes we move to the recognition, following William James (1890/1950, cited in Johnson 2007, p. 94), that 'in all our thinking, we are in some degree aware, however vaguely, of our bodily states, as they result from our interactions in the world' (Johnson 2007, pp. 94–95). Meaning 'is grounded in bodily experience; it arises from our feeling of qualities, sensory patterns, movements, changes and emotional contours' (Johnson 2007, p. 70). Moreover, 'Before and beneath reflective thinking and inquiry, our world stands forth qualitatively' (Johnson 2007, p. 94).

For Gendlin (1997, p. 96, original emphasis) bodily knowledge is beneath and before *perception*:

> The bodily tissue-process we feel (are, speak from ...) is an *immediate* environmental interaction even without perceptions. It is only elaborated by perception and language. We live immediately in our situations; we physically breathe, digest, get angry, or cry. Our words come *immediately* from (and are part of) living in the situation. So we don't want to fall back into the old assumption that the world we live in is only *presented before us*, only perceived and observed, only signalled from the outside.

What does this idea of embodied understanding mean in relation to our analysis of Fit to Drive? People are constantly involved in thinking, perceiving, constructing concepts, reflecting. Whether they are moving, placed in a different physical space, or sitting quietly listening to a story or watching a film. Their embodied experience of the 'flow of meaning making' will have a particular quality in this context. Is it significant that – or whether – Fit to Drive incorporates various sensory, physical and aesthetic means to appeal to and stimulate young people? Traditional representational theories of mind, which treat concepts and thoughts as abstract structures – 'quasi-objects' (Johnson 2007, p. 117) would accord little, if any, significance to the embodied experience of the workshop participants. But if we accept that thinking flows from and within 'patterns of organism–environment coupling' (ibid.), and that there is a complex relationship 'between the lived body, the life-world, and language' (Todres 2007, p. 2) then the qualitative nature of the situation in which a new insight is formed acquires a particular significance.

This chapter explores the facilitated small group workshop – a staple element of much youth work, and much health promotion with young people. The activities in the small group are designed to stimulate young people to think about questions of driving and driving culture in the context of their values and beliefs about driving, and to re-frame their thinking in light of the ideas and challenges they encounter during the morning's workshop. Their experience in the small group is an essential element of this process. The specific task, or intent, in the workshop groups is to generate new knowledges about road safety. This chapter begins to explore the means by which the workshop groups work to enable young people to rethink their orientation to road safety in the light of new information, exploration of values, and engagement with others. It also considers the role and practice of the facilitator in creating the conditions for young people to rethink their attitudes and beliefs in relation to road use.

A particular interest in exploring the 'qualitative nature of the situation' frames our discussion here. We are interested in identifying and exploring the structure, pace and rhythm of small group encounters – the way they 'work'. That is, how the activities are conducted, how they flow, what it is the facilitators do, the place – and the 'work' – of the students. Reference to writers in phenomenological traditions allows us to explore the relationship between thought/language and bodies/movement, and embodied meaning making in the small group workshop setting. Meaning, we will argue, comes into being in the textured experiencing of the 'physical, biological, social, embodied, world' (Johnson 2007, p. 94). Meaning is interactional, and part of the process of experiencing (Gendlin 1962). The interaction occurs not just at the level of the embodied self, but also with/within the social world. Embodied meaning making is inter-relational and inter-subjective, and, in this sense, is always present in health promotion interventions, but often little recognised, little emphasised within the limits of reasoned, rational decision making paradigms.

In the chapter we will describe what happens throughout the various workshop activities, and analyse young people's participation in the workshop session, as well as the role and practice of the facilitator, to explore the realm of dialogue, and of language in these types of encounter. We also consider how ideas, thoughts, feelings, reason and rationality are expressed within the physical space of the workshop (emphasising movement, bodies and energy).

To illustrate the facilitated group-learning environment that is established in the first small group workshop, we describe in detail the first two activities of the workshop, an introductory ice-breaker, and the development of a group agreement. The activities that follow these in the session (which aren't reproduced here, though we will refer to them in our discussion) are 'Choose your activity', a hypothetical that requires young people to choose between three 'risky' activities and discuss the reasons for their decision, and a 'Values' discussion activity in which the students are asked to share their views on statements relating to driving and other road use situations.

Do …

The group session takes place in a smallish, but bright, warm and, importantly, carpeted room in the arts block.[2]

Once in the room the facilitator, Marnie, gets a couple of students to help move the tables to create an open space. She instructs the students to write their names on a sticky label. Once that's done she greets the group and introduces herself. 'Hello, my name is Marnie and I'll be your facilitator for today.' She is around 22, with a laconic, relaxed style, but at the same time confident and authoritative. Her manner is friendly, her voice projects clearly into the room, and conveys the expectation that the students will listen and be ready to follow her lead.

To begin the session Marnie asks the students to stand in a circle, joining them in the circle herself: 'A nice, tight circle. ... You guys all know each other and I'm not that scary, I think.' (laughter) 'Well, I hope not. Alright, how're we going, girls?' (to the girls giving around name stickers and pens) 'You might have to push these chairs out of the way. Come in guys, so you can see each other. Alright!' She checks again that the students' name tags are visible.

Marnie holds up a green tennis ball, saying: 'As you can see I'm holding a tennis ball in my hand. I'm going to throw it to Sally, as I say her name. She's going to throw it to someone else saying their name, and so on, and so on until the ball is thrown around the circle, everyone has received the ball once and it is returned to me. Two things you have to remember: who you received the ball from and who you are throwing the ball to. Any questions?'

There's mainly good humoured interest, smiles, anticipation, rubbing hands, shuffling, particularly from the boys. The girls are more reserved, waiting quietly. Marnie throws the ball to a girl opposite her, calling out her name, 'Sally!' Sally catches the ball, searches for someone to throw to, calls their name, and the ball is off around the group, with the students calling out names as they throw. After the ball has gone around the whole group Marnie repeats the process with the one ball a couple of times. On the third round she introduces another ball to the process, then starts throwing the remaining tennis balls into the group in rapid succession, calling out Sally's name each time. The balls end up flying around the group chaotically. There's laughter, squeals, shouts, calls as the students try to catch and return the ever-increasing numbers of balls being thrown into the group. Marnie cautions the group: 'Nice and gentle.'

The activity has broken the reserve of the girls, and they are fully participating in the game, laughing, engaging in good-natured teasing. More laughter, shouts, confusion. It gets noisier as names are being called. Balls are shooting across the room, and students struggle, and fail, to keep up. After a few minutes of this, Marnie starts collecting all the balls into the bag as each one returns to her. She puts down the bag and returns to the circle, asking: 'How did you feel doing this activity?' A few of the students offer: 'Fun.' 'Confused.' 'Chaotic.' 'Difficult.' Marnie draws out further responses with more specific questions: 'Guys, how did it feel with only one ball?' 'Pretty easy,' the students respond. 'Then with many balls?' 'Confusing', 'Hectic', 'He tried to kill me!' are among the confusion of comments that come back.

Marnie continues in this vein, drawing out the students' experience during the activity. 'So, two or more became difficult? And what happened when we threw them all in?' 'Anything else? Did you find that a bit challenging?' She continues the de-brief by questioning, summarising and paraphrasing the responses. 'I sort of got the impression that there were a lot of balls under the table. When it was getting difficult, I got the impression you started using some strategies to keep it on track. Yeah? Did anyone use any strategies?' Marnie draws out and explores the responses, paraphrasing and checking she's captured the student's meaning. 'Yep, so focussing on that person?' 'Did you try any other strategies? Watched the person who was throwing it to you. So, anticipating, yeah?' … 'So, as the difficulties increased, strategies were being developed to do it more effectively?'

After exploring some of the strategies Marnie asks the students: 'So what do you think this activity might be about? What do we think these tennis balls represent?' A couple of wags reply: 'Ball handling skills.' 'Throwing' …

Marnie: 'Yeah, what else apart from throwing and catching?'

Students start to offer replies that connect the activity with driving: 'Driving a car on the road … Other cars … passengers … More than one car … Pedestrians … Radio …Cyclists … Weather … Hail.' (laughter at this last) Marnie responds to these suggestions with paraphrasing, or affirmations: 'Yeah, absolutely … yeah, good one.'

One student eventually comes up with the suggestion, 'Distractions' and the group builds on this idea: 'Distractions inside and outside the car. Anything's that moving outside.'

Marnie: 'What's the big one nowadays?' A student, quick as a whip: 'Trucks!' (laughter), then, more seriously, 'Mobile phones.'

Marnie brings the activity to a close. She draws the parallels between the activity and driving, concluding with the statement: 'So driving is a complex task. So maybe, when you're driving, a strategy might be to focus, to anticipate what's coming and to focus on what you're doing. Because there are going to be a lot of distractions both inside and outside the car.'

Having finished the activity, Marnie invites the students to sit down. The students, still laughing and joking, arrange themselves around the room, sitting on desks against the walls. Marnie moves to the back of the room and attaches a piece of butcher's paper to the back wall. She calls for a volunteer to scribe. There's some 'volunteering' between the students until a female student (Sally) jumps up to volunteer. She takes the butcher's paper back to where she's sitting on the table, bending to write on the table top as the guidelines are suggested.

Marnie, sitting informally on the floor at the front (body language indicating her 'giving over/handing back' power to the group), sets the scene: 'So, one thing I've noticed already is this room's quite small and it tends to echo quite a bit so what we're going to do right now is just spend a minute creating some guidelines. I don't like the word "rules" because that's sort of, me telling you … So, I want you to come up with some guidelines that you would like, just for this day, just for the two sessions, how you would like it to run, just so you can get something out of it. So, what might help, considering the nature of the room?' (as students hesitate) 'What's something we could do?' It takes a moment or two before they seem to feel more comfortable with expressing their ideas, and there is some joking and teasing between some of the boys. Early suggestions include 'One person speaking at a time,' and 'Don't laugh if someone says something that could be serious.'

'Yeah? Sort of give them some respect … So we've got …' (Marnie appears to be both affirming the contributions and getting some structure on the

exercise by recapping the points of agreement) '... paying people respect by listening to them. One person speaking at a time.'

With quite a bit of prompting/pushing – 'Come on guys, what's important to you?' – the group continues to offer suggestions, which Marnie repeats for the scribe to write up as a list on the butcher's paper. Though she encourages the scribe (and the group) to 'use your own words' she does quite a bit of interpreting, re-framing, clarifying.

Sometimes Marnie re-frames the suggestions, it seems, for clarity or brevity. Sometimes it involves a slight shift to encompass a more general idea. Such as 'giving them respect'.

Marnie gets Sally to read out the agreement from the list she has written down. 'Good, fine. I'm going to give you some blue tack and you can put that up.' She makes a final check with the group. 'Are we happy with these?'

'Can we add to them as we go on?' asks one student. Marnie affirms that this is OK, and finishes the activity by noting that they will aim to stick to the agreement throughout the morning.

'*Do then talk*' is Bern's instruction to the facilitators in training. This phrase, which, in its constant repetition has become almost a mantra, captures ideas about 'discovery learning' that are embedded in the facilitated group approach. The priority is to get the students immediately into the activities, to get them moving, thinking and talking. If a facilitator does too much talking at the beginning of an activity this negates the 'discovery' effect of the exercise. It is in the subsequent 'talk' following the activity that the learning is imagined as occurring. Marnie's first words, after briefly introducing herself, are connected with arranging the space (moving tables if necessary) and the students in the space: 'a nice, tight, circle'. Close together, establishing (physical) connection, and then immediately into the instructions for the tennis ball activity. The key is to get the energy going, and students into the 'moment'. The activity is both an 'ice-breaker' – as the name implies, a method of dispelling group members' natural reserve and reluctance to participate – and an immediate entrée into the topic. The tennis balls have become symbolically important in the workshop, and both facilitators and presenters have adopted the practice of linking back to the 'tennis balls' to symbolise driving distractions. Facilitators will talk of 'tennis balls happening in the room', if they want to draw attention to distracting or disruptive behaviour in the group.

Deceptively simple, the tennis ball activity becomes very confusing if the facilitators ramble, forget key points, backtrack and prolong the introduction. The beginning has to be clear and simple with a planned descent into chaos as students start to experience the impossibility of keeping up with all the balls being thrown into the circle. Instructions are tightly scripted, and are kept to the most basic. They have been refined over a number of years to keep the 'wordiness' to a minimum, to avoid facilitators waffling and sapping energy from the activity, and therefore the group.

The relationship between doing and talking, the interconnection and interplay of language and bodily presence/movement, lies at the heart of the small group experience. This applies equally to the facilitator and the group participants. The role of the facilitator in the workshops is, essentially, to create the conditions for the young people to become actively involved in the construction of meaning and the building of (new) knowledges about driving, road use, risk and being safe. As the facilitator training notes observe, the requirement of facilitation is

> fundamentally … to engage the group members in a very short time and encourage participation in a variety of forms. Responding to the group is the key aspect here. The activities are tools for the facilitators to engage and encourage participation.
>
> (Ariens 2007, p. 1)

Participation of the young people is signalled by the verbal: talking, affirming, challenging, clarifying, questioning; and the non-verbal: listening, reflecting, imagining, being 'present', doing (the activities). For the facilitator the task is to create a safe space to move the students through a process of reflection, triggered by the activities, and the development of new understandings about themselves in relation to road safety. This is most obviously achieved through the medium of language: through the discussion, questioning, clarifying and provision of information that occurs in the context of the activities. But in focussing on language as the fundamental key to understanding the workshops and what it is the facilitators do, it is easy to overlook the physical dimension of the experience – the body in the workshop space. Any observation of the Fit to Drive facilitators at work affirms that what they do is very much grounded in the physical 'being in the space' as well as what is said in that space. Facilitation is very much about 'performance'. This encompasses the way they move around the workshop room, their gestures, stance and positioning while they listen, affirm, draw out, or alternatively, close off, discussion.

The physical arrangement and disposition of the students in the space – high energy in the first activity (ice-breaker), through to more quietly reflective in the group agreement – is signalled by the demeanour, the 'presence' of the facilitator. To introduce the group agreement Marnie sits on the floor. This can be read on one level as a democratic act, indicating the 'giving over', or sharing, of her power in the group. At the same time it is the action of a group leader who is in control of the situation, and what's happening in the group. Importantly, it signals a change of pace, a new orientation in the group dynamic.

In training Bern draws attention to the importance of the body in facilitating, focussing on gestures, positioning in relation to the group, 'open/closed' bodily signals, eye contact. The facilitator can signal inclusiveness, capture – and show – attention, settle restless behaviour by, for example, a change of position in relation to the group, a sweep of the arm, becoming still, making eye contact, by shepherding the students into small groups. The physicality is important to the workshop experience in fundamental ways. It is there in the placement of bodies, in the way the young people group themselves, make themselves comfortable and settle into the room. It is there the moment the facilitator enters the room and arranges the layout. The way the facilitator and young people connect. How they 'meet in the space'. In the 'choreography' of the activities.

For many years when we taught group work to undergraduate youth work students we found it useful to draw on the idea of 'choreography' as a way of prompting them to think through their actions and movement when planning and preparing for a group session. By this we meant the practical step-by-step sequence of activities, the timing, the arrangement of bodies. For the purpose of visualising the 'performance zone', the people in the group were a 'mass' occupying the space. Students were encouraged to include in their planning a mental picture of the group, themselves in relation to the group, where they would place the participants, the arrangement of seating, or floor space for sitting, where and when they would move, change position and how they would manage the physical movement from one activity to the next. The reference to 'choreography' was practical, designed to convey to the students the idea of planning for group work that incorporated an awareness of timing and placement. At the same time this attention to movement, the use of space and the general physicality of group work also point to the deeper meaning and place of the body in that process. The relationship between the bodily experience – the physical – and the intellectual processing of the workshop is intricately woven. The significance of the body in the workshop space is about more than the 'learning by doing' of kinaesthetic learning. It is about the nature of the 'felt experience', or the 'felt quality' of the situation that is fundamental to meaning making.

… then talk

Ultimately, it is 'talk' that is seen to be the main business of the Fit to Drive workshops. It is understood that through 'talk' new knowledges relating to driving and road use are constructed: through the imparting and sharing of information, discussion of feelings, values, experiences and opinions. The workshops are designed to work with the explicit expression of feelings, prejudices, values, opinions, facts. In this sense, the 'conversations' enacted in the workshops continue a process of socialisation, in Gadamer's (2006, p. 548) sense: 'we learn a language and grow into everything we learn by way of conversation. This is the process that is nowadays called "socialisation" – growth into the social'.

This is exemplified in the group agreement. The group agreement is a standard strategy in group work practice for establishing group norms in relation to conduct and interaction between group members (Douglas 1991; Johnson and Johnson 2003). It is both preventative of problems in the group and productive, in that it contributes to group building, and focuses the group members on the task and the promotion of positive communication. Facilitators usually engage one of the students to write up the agreement as a way of emphasising that it is to be 'owned' by the group, not something imposed by the facilitators as quasi-teachers.

The group agreement, ideally, is the beginning of a conversation. And group facilitation in a learning environment may be viewed as fostering an extended conversation. Drawing on Gadamer (2006, p. 387), it is the start of a process, through language, of coming to an understanding, of opening up the possibilities of the emergence of something new: 'it belongs to every true conversation that each person opens himself to the other'. Therefore, the group agreement must establish a 'safe' environment in which each young person may feel supported to 'open themselves up' to the other.

There is always the danger that the process of coming to a group agreement can become a token exercise – most students will be at least familiar with, socialised into, the idea. The skill of the facilitator is to move beyond token, though perhaps sincere, responses such as 'listening', 'respect', 'one person talking at a time', to a more meaningful exploration of the nature of communication, connection and valuing others. Facilitators, and sometimes students in the group, will make reference to the group agreement as a way of reminding other students of the expectation that the right to speak, and be heard – to *participate in the conversation* – is one that has been established as part of the *common ground*. 'Finding a common language is not … preparing a tool for the purpose of reaching understanding' observes Gadamer (2006, p. 389), 'but, rather, coincides with the very act of understanding and reaching agreement'. Formation of understanding (meaning) occurs socially, *through* language. For Gadamer (2006, p. 390): 'language is the form in which understanding is achieved'. People come to *know* through the act of speaking. Even thought – internalised speech – is conversation with the imagined other.

If language is a primary means for achieving understanding, this occurs in a 'shared world of culture and language' according to Todres (2007, p. 16), that then 'shows itself as a central feature in the drama of understanding'. The language created in the group for the purposes of conducting the conversation around driving and road use draws on a common fund of concepts and language, and a common culture. For Kenan Malik (2000, p. 332), in his study of theories of the human mind, 'language is a thread that links a particular human individual to other human individuals, both past and present'. Malik explores the idea of the 'extended mind' – the idea that the human mind is shaped, and comes into being, within a specifically social context, and through social interaction. Meaning is socially constructed: 'the mind is not just a private but also a social phenomenon … it is best understood in terms of a set of relationships between the individual and the social, cultural and historical networks he [sic] inhabits' (Malik 2000, p. 334). Each young person experiencing Fit to Drive does so in the context of their own experience and understanding. In Graham's words, 'their own personal journey'.

At the same time we must acknowledge post-structuralist insights that language and conversation and discursive practices always involve a struggle over meaning. Power relations, gender, class and ethnic relations, the histories of young people's involvement in processes and practices of school-based meaning making, are all at play in these sorts of group encounters. Language is never neutral or transparent. Its differing opacity is evident in the limited struggle by Marnie to 'facilitate' the setting of the rules of engagement for these sessions.

An important feature of language is that it is also *creative* of understanding. Understanding occurs through the search for expression of felt experience, semi-formed ideas, hunches. It occurs, moreover, through the process of 'troubling', or unsettling, previously unexamined or taken-for-granted thinking. This is achieved (or at least aimed for) in the workshop activities that involve the participants in expressing – 'giving voice' to – opinions, beliefs and values. Todres (2007, p. 16) explores the element of 'adventure' that is involved in Gadamer's notion of understanding. For Gadamer (2006, p. xvii), understanding requires participants in the 'conversation' to be willing to open themselves 'to the emergence of something else, the … subject matter that comes to presence and presentation in conversation'. This process, the coming to understanding through language, involves an element of 'moving forward': 'speaking is only speaking if we accept the risk of positing something and following out its implications' (Gadamer 2006, p. 553). In the small group workshop the task for the group members is to offer thoughts, ideas, opinions, questions, and to follow these ideas, to 'explore' them in the new terrain that has come into being through not only language, but also through the staging, the space and the embodied experience. The experience allows for the emergence of 'something else'. It is a movement forward to a new understanding.

The idea of understanding-as-movement appears in various metaphorical forms in the phenomenological tradition. In Chapter 5 we explore Husserl's conceptualisation of understanding as a movement that proceeds from a 'home' towards the 'other'. Imagined as journey, from a metaphorical 'home', there is a play of tension between the familiar 'homeworld' and the unfamiliar 'alien' (Todres 2007, p. 15). Todres (2007, p. 16) refers to the movement towards understanding as a 'productive tension between appropriation and transgression', a movement that is suggestive of Gadamer's idea of the 'risk' of exploring the 'implications' of what will come into being in the process (of becoming language). This is a risk that is inherent in the small group sessions, in the commitment to opening up the process and to work with what the students 'discover' in the facilitated discussions. In Fit to Drive, the group agreement, in essence, must establish the 'ground' for this to occur. The conversations generated by the activities in the small group may require of the students that they 'move out of their comfort zone' – an overused term in popular psychology that nevertheless carries interesting resonances of the philosophical idea of understanding as movement from 'home'.

The idea of 'emergence' – Gadamer's 'emergence of something else' – brings us back to an awareness of the fluid, embodied, nature of understanding.

Language grows out of, and around, the embodied act/process of meaning making. The task of the facilitators is, partly, to be midwife to the words, to the language that may transform understanding, and be creative of new understanding/s; to coax into being the language that will be shared in that specific space/time.

Silence has its own quality and is imbued with significance. Facilitators are trained to pick up on silence – especially if it is interpreted as expressive silence – and to draw this out to become language – to achieve an understanding. In the process of young people's articulation of their unspoken feelings, responses and (unformed) thoughts, there is a coming to, or movement towards, understanding, for the young person, and for others in the conversation.

Body and language: partners in a conversation

Body and language, as 'partners in a conversation', come together in the participatory and experiential learning that occurs in the small groups. This is an important part of the aesthetic dimension of the Fit to Drive workshop experience. This includes the quality of experience, bodily responses to situations, the felt sense of situations. It thus also extends to the notion of 'aesthetics' in the more generally understood sense of the word – the interest, novelty, drama, visual effect: the appeal to senses. Meaning starts here.

It is in this sort of context that Todres (2007, p. 35) explores the implications of Gendlin's description of knowing as 'both an embodied and languaged process'. Gendlin emphasises the interrelationship of language and bodily experience – language is an embodied, physical act. Todres (2007, p. 33) explains that, for Gendlin:

> language and bodily experience cannot simply be reduced to one another – both require one another as partners in a conversation, and both phases (embodying and languaging) constitute both limits and freedoms in this conversation – hopefully, a productive tension. Sometimes, the bodily depth of what one has lived through is 'more than words can say'. Yet such experience 'looks for' words.

In this context, language includes non-verbal means of expression and understanding, such as dance. 'What Gendlin calls the "linguistic" pertains to all forms of symbolic interaction, from music to painting to dance to ritual to gesture to sign language' (Johnson 2007, p. 83). Johnson draws attention to the place of Gendlin's work in alerting us to the importance of 'our felt sense of the situation out of which meaning and thought emerge' (Johnson 2007, p. 84). For Gendlin (1991) concepts have a felt meaning. It is to the meaning associated with the felt sense of the thought or idea that we return as we try to articulate the thought, to express it, or put it into words. Here Gadamer (2006, p. 552) suggests that language is a visceral experience, an act of 'taking a word into your mouth'.

In the discussion following each activity the facilitator seeks to draw out the reactions, thoughts and views of the students. A student offers an opinion, or relates an experience: 'Tell me more about that,' prompts the facilitator. 'Why do you think that is?' as they encourage the student to follow the trail of her thought, to capture her idea. The student may be on a roll, may feel comfortable continuing this line of thought. Or she may hesitate, search, try to pin down the 'full sense' of what she wants to express. Her 'felt sense' of the situation (Gendlin 1995; Johnson 2007). The ease, or unease, that she feels. The emotions, the bodily sensations attached here are a conduit for reflection, and for understanding, limited or otherwise.

For Johnson (2007), logical relations are felt, not just thought. An interruption in the flow of thought, a failure to grasp something, or struggle to express something, to 'think the thought', will be experienced as a feeling of bodily discomfort, being stuck. The first question the facilitator asks when the tennis balls have been collected and the group is settled in the circle is: 'How do you feel?' Feeling is the primary experience. Meaning comes into being within that primary experience. The question captures them within the moment/presence of that experience.

In the small group workshop 'Marnie' had invited 'Roland' to talk about why he moved away from his choice in the 'Choose your activity' segment. Roland responds: 'You feel safe if you're driving with Mum or Dad. Driving with Mum and Dad is …' he trails off, as he appears to struggle to complete his thought. Marnie interprets Roland's meaning: 'So there's confidence in the familiar.' 'Yeah' says Roland. Here, possibly, it might have been more appropriate for the facilitator to delve a little deeper into the meaning of what 'feel safe' meant for Roland. What is the quality of the experience he was describing as 'feeling safe'? Before Roland has had the chance to put the feeling into words – he seems to have a definite 'felt sense' of what this means, and discover for himself what it is that makes him feel safe – the facilitator has provided an interpretation, which Roland has agreed with, and the conversation moves on. As with much, if not all, small group type encounters between young people and facilitators (teachers, workers) in institutional settings the facilitator is juggling a number of imperatives: awareness of time constraints, allowing others to speak, the task of pulling together and summarising the content of the discussion, and guiding the discussion to a point where the hoped for, preferred meanings come into focus and can be shaped into clear educational messages.

The understanding of meaning making and knowing developed within phenomenological traditions may (also) provide an insight into the more fundamental role of the facilitator in the workshop. In this context Todres' (2007, p. 35) interest in Gendlin's concept of situated meaning is useful. Gendlin, for whom meanings of a situation are 'more than words can say', refers to a 'preseparated multiplicity' to describe the 'felt sense' of meaning that is present 'prior to logical, conceptual organisation': '[L]ogic works only with what has been separated. But a situation is a preseparated multiplicity and carrying it forward opens up new possibilities that were not separately there before' (Gendlin 1991, cited in Todres, 2007, p. 33). At one level the facilitator's role may be expressed in terms of creating the space for the students to identify, express, and explore their values, thoughts and opinions about road safety. From a phenomenological perspective the role takes on a deeper dimension. The task of the facilitator in the workshop is to assist the students to locate, and give expression to, the felt sense of their understanding of their experience, or situation. To assist in separating the 'preseparated multiplicity' of their experience. This involves bringing the language into being that will carry forward the 'felt experience' of what they are trying to express. To become concepts, ideas, and descriptions while paying attention to the felt sense of what the words are attempting to capture. 'Moving forward' is a metaphorical description that also refers to the bodily sense of this experience. Johnson (2007, p. 95, original emphasis) expands on the idea of 'felt sense' – 'the way it feels to think the thoughts' – and links this to the idea of thought as 'flowing'. 'Since *thought flows*, there must be a quality of this flow that we can experience'. There is an embodied process of felt movement, of change. Indeed, 'our reflections are carried out in the temporal flux on which we are trying to seize' (Merleau-Ponty 2008, p. xv). Words themselves contain particular felt qualities. For instance, 'if' carries a sense of 'anticipation of something that follows, in a way that moves you to a new thought-location' (Johnson 2007, p. 95). The words 'if … then' in that particular grammatical construction, are imbued with a certain quality: 'if' with a sense of anticipation; 'then' carrying the feeling of resolution, settlement. The 'felt quality' of a word can, then, convey a sense of movement forward.

In the facilitator training program the complex practice of group facilitation has been condensed into a number of key learnings and principles, to bring the trainees to a initial level of competence in facilitation. These key points are a blend of description (of what facilitators do) and principles. From practical guidelines ('Do then talk'), to more complex skills, such as reflective listening. Each is a shorthand description of an aspect of facilitation that encompasses theory and subtleties of practice, and Bern elaborates on these (within the limits of the available training time). One of 'Bern's rules' is 'Get rid of the "but"'. As an example, discussing the process of 'validating' individual students by paraphrasing their contribution, Bern describes what happens when the word 'but' is used to move the conversation along. 'Thank you for your thoughts, Briony, *but* we'd like to hear from Jacinta …' What Bern has highlighted is the feeling that is attached to the word 'but': it conveys the sense of negating the validation that had occurred through the facilitator's reflective listening and paraphrasing:

> There is not a conjunction or a preposition, and hardly an adverbial phrase, syntactic form, or inflection of voice, in human speech, that does not express some shading or other of relation which we at some moment actually feel to exist between the larger objects of our thought …

> We ought to say a feeling of *and*, a feeling of *if*, a feeling of *but*, and a feeling of *by*, quite as readily as we say a feeling of *blue* or a feeling of *cold*.
> (James 1890/1950, 1:245–246, cited in Johnson 2007, p. 96)

'But' has a very specific felt meaning. In a chapter titled, with a knowing wink, 'Feeling William James's "But"', Johnson observes that, to 'feel James's "but" is to feel the quality of a situation as a kind of hesitancy or qualification of a something asserted or proposed' (Johnson 2007, p. 96). What Bern has been alert to, is the 'felt sense' conveyed by words, syntax and expression, and the way this will influence what the young person feels, their sense of feeling listened to, or not; and, ultimately, how this will impact on their learning.

In this discussion we have drawn on philosophical understandings that recognise language as *generative* of knowledge and meaning making. The act of producing, and sharing language, moreover, constitutes an event experienced in the workshop: 'language is not an entity, but something that inheres in the act of utterance and thus becomes an event, something historical' (Gadamer 2006, p. 394). It is where the young people and the Fit to Drive program (with all this implies) meet: a 'happening', in the sense of an event/experience that is transformative for the participants, and the space itself. When, as will often occur, a teacher looks in the window during the workshop to check on the group, she is able to make an assessment of the energy and feel of the room by observation alone. The space (the atmosphere, the energy, the feel of the bodies in the space) has been transformed. The language that has comes into being in the workshop space has contributed to the transformation of that space.

To grasp the transformative nature of the learning that occurs in the facilitated learning activities, we must also turn to understandings of meaning making that comprehend the fundamentally aesthetic, embodied nature of this process. If meaning is 'assembled' in the group 'encounter' (Gubrium and Holstein 2009) this occurs within a dynamic flow of meaning making that is deeply rooted in the aesthetic, bodily experience of being part of this grouping in this space.

Central to the transformative potential of the learning that occurs in the small group is the skill of the facilitator. At a most basic level this involves a complex of skills: to paraphrase what group members have said; to ask open rather than closed questions; to keep discussion on track; to summarise the main points; and to tie this in to the themes and road safety messages. Further skill – and judgement – is required to involve quiet group members, to probe deeper, to 'get to the bottom' of participants' opinions and ideas, feelings and intuitions. At times the facilitators have to judge when it's appropriate and necessary to change the approach, or strategy, and to adapt it to meet the requirements of the group. The skill and expertise of the facilitators, the best of whom display the level of artistry that Bourdieu (1990) refers to as 'virtuosity' or 'feel for the game', are the key to the creation of the space in which new knowledges are generated (see also Healy 1994; Flyvbjerg 2006).

John Law (2004) argues for method assemblages that can encounter and acknowledge and work and play with different ways of knowing. This call is not abstract, disembodied, removed from different contexts. What it gestures towards are multiplicities and emergent ways of knowing. In the contexts we have been discussing here, settings that are widespread and familiar in an array of ways of working with young people in schools and elsewhere, we have tried to make present the embodied, the aesthetic dimensions of meaning making. Small group encounters, as educational and work practices, necessarily assemble diverse actors in spaces and processes that are up-close-and-personal. Part of our purpose here, the 'good' we are trying to produce, is to make apparent the limits and possibilities of thinking if we continue to work with ideas that privilege particular understandings of reason and rationality as being somehow disembodied, as being located largely in an individual's cognitive capacities. Understood in these ways, cognitive capacities for reason and rationality promise to tame the emotional, the embodied, the aesthetic dimensions of the ways in which we apprehend and make sense of the world.

The challenge, as we see it, is to open up these sorts of small group assemblages, and our ways of interpreting, analysing and critiquing them, to the felt senses of uncertainty, ambiguity, ambivalence and emergence that we have made present in this discussion. In returning to a theme, in many of the settings and spaces where these assemblages emerge, are formed, these felt senses are troubling and unsettling. They trouble and unsettle the school day. The need to accommodate a timetable. Time. Relationships. Facilitation. Curriculum and pedagogy. The demands for a degree of enclosure. 'Goods'. What remains most unsettling may be the trouble we continue to have with bodies. Young bodies in particular. A troubling that is made a little clearer with the sense that 'her body thinks …'

Notes

1 The Monavale case study is described in detail in Chapter 6.
2 Madderlake College first small group session.

5 'What happened was this ... '

What roles do stories have in health promotion?

The lights dim, and the film Birthday *('a film by Shannon Sleith') appears on the screen. The film opens on a recognisable scene: a birthday party – perhaps a twenty-first – held in the rumpus room of a suburban family home, decorated in shades of brown, trophies, photos, a bar. A mix of friends and family gather to hear the traditional speech; smiles greet the best friend of the 'birthday boy' as he gets up to speak. The Friend launches into a light hearted, mocking, birthday speech. As the smiles and laughter of the gathered friends continue, the tone becomes eerie, and the sound track strikes an ominous note. The speaker's smiles and jokes fade, for now he is hesitating, and turning to his friend, he says: 'But as they say, all good things must come to an end, because – later on tonight – I'm going to kill him.' More laughter from the gathered friends and family. There are mixed reactions from the workshop audience – gasps of shock, some laughter. The Friend, shaking himself out of his sombre mood, smiles, presses on. 'So, while I'm up here I thought it was fitting that I should tell you a little about the man, after all, this will be the last time any of you will see David alive.'* [1]

We have argued that the emotional dimensions of the Fit to Drive workshops are essential to the engagement of the young people in the problem of road safety. The fundamental technique of appeal to the emotions is through the medium of story. In the opening segment of many of the workshops, Graham's (the workshop presenter) self-deprecating humour generates a level of emotional empathy in the group, and elicits the goodwill to pay attention to the story that immediately follows, the affecting 'Julie's Story'. The commencement of Julie's story heralds a tonal shift in the workshop, when the students are confronted with the reality of the business of the day – road crashes and their prevention. It is through this story that the emotional connection with the problem of road safety is established. With the words *'What I want to do is capture the moment, though, when my life changed'*, Graham signals the start of the story with a classic storytelling 'hook'. As the story unfolds it brings together some of the themes for the day: inexperience, managing distractions on the roads and in the car, peer influence, consequences of crashes. Like the other stories it is a fundamentally cautionary tale. The message: 'It can happen to anybody', aims to counteract the pervasive 'It won't happen to me' belief held by many or all of us, most or all of the time.

Stories, many of them powerful and affecting, are at the heart of Fit to Drive. Facts and rational arguments are the 'nuts and bolts', the recognisable 'moving parts' of the system. But stories are the fuel, propelling the enterprise and igniting the imagination and understanding of the audience. The stories are big and small. Sacred, communal 'Fit to Drive' stories told and refined over time, and personal, individual narratives contributing in both acknowledged and unseen ways to the fabric of the program. Each Fit to Drive story, in its telling, reflects a differently nuanced point of reference to think through the problem of young people and road trauma.

Within the first 10–15 minutes of the workshop the young people are told three stories. One is 'Julie's Story', which recounts the events that originally activated Graham's involvement in road safety education, and became the catalyst for the development of Fit to Drive. 'Julie's Story' is in fact intertwined with 'Graham's Story', and the story of the journey to 'find an answer' to young driver crashes. The second story is told in a short film; the story of a young man who is responsible for the death of his best friend in a car crash. The third is offered as background to the short film. It is the story of the young film-maker who wrote and directed the film after losing her friends in a crash. Other stories follow in later segments of the workshop. The Australian Rules footballer David Hille tells, in a filmed interview, of the events leading to the crash he was involved in that claimed two lives and injured others. The Metropolitan Fire Brigade Monavale case study depicts a complex and dramatic story that forms the basis for an extended group discussion session in the workshop. Other case scenarios build stories in which students create and enact their own endings. Alongside these stories are those of the workshop participants – students, facilitators and presenters. Some will be told in the course of the workshop, some will remain unspoken but will be, often powerfully, present for each person.

In Chapter 2 we referenced James Wood's (2008) examination of how fiction works, and his claim that we can explore the workings of fiction by letting go of a sense that fiction references 'the real', and by taking up the possibilities of the profound 'truthfulness' of fiction. To recap, Wood (2008, pp. 178–179) argues that 'the question of fiction's referentiality – does fiction make true statements about the world? – is the wrong one, because fiction does not ask us to believe things (in a philosophical sense) but to imagine them (in an artistic sense)'. In this way, imagining 'the heat of the sun on your back is about as different an activity as can be from believing that tomorrow it will be sunny. One experience is all but sensual, the other wholly abstract'. And so, as we discussed earlier, when we encounter a variety of texts, representations, stories, fictions, we can stumble upon what Wood (2008, p. 184) calls the 'blue river of truth': the space in which we might engage 'scenes and moments and perfectly placed words in fiction and poetry, in film and drama, which strike us with their truth, which move and sustain us, which shake habits' house to its foundations'. While Wood's reference is to debates about fiction and its relation to the 'real', his comments about the aesthetic dimensions of the work that fiction, that stories, can do – the work of meaning making, is important to the things that we want to discuss in this chapter. Particularly as many of the stories that give structure to the flow and work of this health promotion intervention are 'fictionalised' accounts of 'real' incidents and crashes. As 'fictions' they are much more than 'factual' accounts of the 'real' events, 'real' crashes.

Our purpose here is to analyse the role of storytelling in the potentially transformative practices of much health promotion with young people. The role of stories in sense making, and the generation of meaning, has been explored by a number of writers (McIntyre 1981; Ochs and Capps 2001; Polkinghorne 1988; Weick 1995). We will draw on this literature to argue that there are profound relations between stories, emotions and morals, that these relations are to be found in much health promotion with young people, and that these relations ought to be made explicit in making sense of the limits and possibilities of these types of interventions. So, we will examine the narrative devices that are a feature of these stories; the impact of 'backshadowing' and 'foreshadowing' the events of the story; the place of myth; and the motif of 'journey' that shape many of the stories that young people encounter in the Fit to Drive workshop. We will also explore the place of personal narrative and examine the ways in which the personal narratives of those who have been affected by road trauma connect with the stories told in Fit-to-Drive.

Birthday and 'Shannon's Story'

Following Julie's story, recounted by the presenter in the opening segment of the workshop, the Traffic Accident Commission (TAC) film *Birthday* is screened.[2] This is the 'fictional' story of David, and his friend, at David's birthday party. Having revealed that later that evening he is going to 'kill him', David's friend continues his speech at the birthday gathering of friends and family:

'For as long as I can remember David he's always lived life to the fullest' (a shot of David, quiet pleasure on his face) 'and in a couple of months he was going to live out his dream, and travel around the world' (the camera captures a smiling, knowing, affectionate glance exchanged between David and a pretty girl with wavy blond hair and a beautiful smile at the front of the crowd).

The Friend becomes sombre. 'Just imagine what you could have seen and done, David.' He gives a serious look to David, then turns to the gathering. 'You know what's really sad about all of this, is that … it doesn't have to happen. I'll be just showing off in front of these guys … (camera pans to close up of two young men, who lift their glasses and give a macho, slightly drunk, cheer in acknowledgement) … taking a few risks on the road.' (close up, showing the Friend taking a reflective pause) 'Well, I suppose I should really try and enjoy this moment because, no-one here is going to look at me in the same way again. Especially his parents.' As he says this he turns, with an expression of sorrow and regret, to David's parents, who are standing at the front of the group with smiles of pride and pleasure. He turns back to David. With the same tone, he asks: 'Good mates are meant to look after their mates, aren't they?' David catches his eye, and looks down, his manner shy, self-effacing, but enjoying the moment. The Friend shakes off the sombre moment and looks up.

Continuing in this vein, he concludes his speech with the presentation of his gift: 'So, before I go I'd just like to give David his last birthday present. It's – ' (he searches in his pocket and pulls out a paper. He shakes the paper nervously, gesturing his reluctance to hand it over) ' – it's your death certificate.' He looks on in numb anxiety as David, smiling, moved by this additional gift and attention, accepts the present. They shake hands. The camera rests on the Friend's face, revealing the emotions struggling there. He is sad, anxious, but he gathers up a smile and turns to the crowd.

'So, let's all raise our glasses, before I end David's life. After all, what are best friends for? To David!' We see David's parents, and the people gathered there, raising their glasses with loving looks, toasting their son, loved one, friend: 'To David!' The last shot is of David's sweet, very young, smiling face, raising his glass in returned salute.

The film closes to a black screen with the words 'a film by Shannon Sleith'.

There is silence as the film fades, the audience still and subdued. During the film there have been some contrasting reactions from the students, although on the whole they have been attentive, their faces serious and focussed on the film. Some of the students have laughed at various points – when the Friend announces he's going to kill his best friend, when the young men at the party – the characters and setting immediately recognisable – raise their glasses and act the fool. As the film's closing lines sink in some draw breath, others laugh awkwardly. The film's black humour with the shock of the line, 'Tonight I'm going to kill him', bitterly uttered by the main character causes a mix of emotional reactions. Most are quiet. Or they gasp in shock when they hear that line.

After a few moments of silence, Graham steps to the front. 'This film was made by Shannon Sleith. Shannon was nineteen years of age when she made this film. She made the film because she was at a party in Gisborne, just outside Melbourne. And at that party, around twelve o'clock – it was a very big party – lots and lots of drinking.' (long pause) 'A group of friends said, lets all go off to Melbourne, roar down the Calder (Freeway), we'll go down to King Street, down to the nightclubs. And Shannon made the decision not to go. She said no I'm not going. The car took off, roared down the highway, and about a kilometre down the highway, swerved into the side of a bridge, and three of her friends were killed. Two ambulance workers who attended that crash never worked again as a result of what they saw.

Graham quietly focuses his attention on the audience, telling the students 'And that film, she made it with what we call black humour, she wanted people to see that this was unbelievable, and to laugh – and I saw the smiles when you suddenly see the death certificate being handed over. She wanted that to happen. She also knew this – that today in this room there will be people in this audience who have been affected by road trauma, there will be people who know, who resonated with that story. And as we move through today, as you make this journey of staying safer, we want you to be very sensitive to just that issue.'

'Graham's Story' and the 'ur-' stories in Fit to Drive

The experience of the loss of so many young lives on the Mornington Peninsula over an eighteen-month period forms the background (genesis) of Fit to Drive. It is the 'ur-story', the story of origin. 'Graham's Story' is just one of the many stories clustered around those events, circumstances and experiences. Any number of principals, teachers, fellow students and friends of any of the fatal crash victims, let alone families and loved ones, would have equally powerful and life-changing stories. However, what we have called 'Graham's Story' contains three stories that belong in the history of Fit to Drive: the story of the young woman killed, ('Julie's Story'), Graham's personal story, and the story of the beginnings of Fit to Drive.

A version of the story is told at the beginning of the workshop at schools on the Peninsula. In other regions the story might be told by another presenter, it may be another story of origin of their own region. Graham's personal narrative has become 'story', and part of Fit to Drive lore. In this sense, Graham himself has become part historical character, as well as current protagonist.

On the other side of the city a school principal in the western region of Melbourne, 'Jim O'Brien', experienced a similar epiphany, and his story has also become part of the Fit to Drive fabric. Jim had lived through a similar experience to Graham, having been principal of a large secondary school in an outer suburb/semi-rural setting. His school community had experienced a spate of crashes that had claimed the lives of students and staff over a period of less than two years. In the workshops he co-ordinates Jim tells of the point when, following yet another funeral, the school chaplain, who had officiated at all the funerals, came to sit with him in his office, finding support together. It was that encounter with the chaplain that Jim identifies as the starting point for his commitment to the promotion of road safety. We heard a version of this story in May 2009:

'Yes – it's a journey; if you'd spoken to me twelve years ago it's a journey I wouldn't have expected to have taken, not in the way I have. The journey came about because, when I was principal at Glencairn Secondary, tragically in 2000, 2001 we had a series of road tragedies which really impacted on the community and impacted on me, involving students, ex-students, and staff, and so I decided in 2001 that I needed to do – I needed maybe to do something about this – and there was a significant moment for me, after the funeral of a year 11 student, we came back – the chaplain that I had at the school took all the funerals, and he and I had developed a close bond with all this – we came back to my office, we sat down and he looked over at me and he said this – you know, significant

words – he said: 'This has got to stop. I don't want to bury any more young people.' So from that day on, he and I, and a local police officer who was working at the school, made an informal pledge – a pledge, but an informal pledge, that we would work in a pro-active way to promote road safety in young people. So, I decided if an opportunity arose – and it did; as a school principal I was always working in proactive ways – but I would like to take this further beyond the Glencairn area. So, I developed a link with VicRoads personnel and others [in the Education Department] – and I decided to take some leave, as school principal, took a term off (unpaid leave) to explore some things, and the next thing I know I was doing some work for the [Traffic Safety Education unit] in road safety as traffic safety coordinator. So, I retired, and took it up in a significant way. That was in 2002. So it's been over six years since I've been doing this sort of work.'

Jim's story, intertwined with 'Shannon's Story', forms another significant anchor point from which to trace the development of Fit to Drive. Jim's story initiated Fit to Drive in the western region of Melbourne, and at the same time helped, continues to help, to give the program in that region its particular character. Jim's story, told at the beginning of the workshops in the west, locates the history strongly in an area that is familiar – 'known' and identified with, lived in – for the audiences, and through identification with familiar territory, and imagined characters, reinforces the impact of the larger Fit to Drive story. The story settings are recognisable to local audiences: the students in the west will be familiar with the rural areas the football team drives through in one of the crashes Jim describes. The audiences in the Peninsula will have a picture in their minds of the coastal bush the young men drive through when they crash into a tree. They will know the road from Frankston to Hastings that Julie drove along, and probably the very roundabout where she crashed. But stories, local or otherwise, are not unproblematic. And we need to develop some sense of storytelling to explore the limits and possibilities of stories in health promotion with young people.

Storytelling, audience and narrative devices

Harold Scheub (1998, p. 3), echoing James Wood, argues that stories 'provide us with truth; they take the flotsam and jetsam of our lives, and give those shards a sense of narrative, of form, and therefore of verity'. In his study of a storytelling tradition Scheub identifies features of storytelling culture and process which are, he claims, common to the storytelling event. In Scheub's account the nature and role of the audience is central to the telling of story. Significantly, audience and teller share a network of images, a prepared ground in which to plant the elements of story. The audience: 'know the narratives of the tradition well; they have the same repertory of inherited images that the artist has, and the artist depends on this. In the storytelling space the audience does more than wordlessly fill in gaps left by the performer; it provides a rich context for the unfolding drama' (Scheub 1998, p. 48).

The relationship between Fit to Drive stories, the teller and their audience mirrors many of the elements of this storytelling tradition. The audience of secondary students know well the narrative traditions at play here. The journey, both actual and symbolic, commenced in great hopefulness and sense of possibility. The tradition of twenty-first birthday celebrations that is depicted in the film *Birthday*; the football team setting off for the game; the students on the last day of school, starting new life adventures; the boys, hopping in the boot of the car with hopes of connecting with the girls that they are attracted to. All these are familiar elements in the stories of young people's lives. The stock of characters is familiar. The storytellers are confident that the familiar settings and events (end of year exams, celebratory party, football match) will resonate with the audience. The individuals in the stories only need to be lightly sketched and the details will be filled in from the audience's shared 'repertory of inherited images'. For many young people in the Fit to Drive audience a certain mythology surrounds the looming last days of school. A mythology that features in Julie's story and other stories in the workshop. This mythology incorporates an assumption of reckless, temporary discarding of responsibilities, abandonment to pleasure, and communal celebration. Other elements of the shared context or tradition that are assumed in the telling of story in Fit to Drive include an awareness of the moral issues at stake, and the ways that they are presented and framed. Some of the values and social expectations reflected in the stories are also familiar and assumed as shared, including 'mateship' and ideas about loyalties within friendship groups.

The combined impact of the stories serves to engage the emotions of the listeners. They provoke/invoke curiosity, empathy, concern. Through the medium of the individual stories told in the introductory session the themes and messages of the workshop are well established, and proceed to form the backdrop for the rest of the workshop program and learning activities to follow in the small groups. The stories are intertwined (Julie/Graham's story; Shannon/'Jim'/'David's Birthday' story; Graham/Jim's intersecting stories) and reinforce the idea of the far-reaching impact of road trauma that is one of the major themes of the Fit to Drive stories.

The telling of Shannon's story places the film in context – as the story of a survivor – and is also a means of debriefing the audience. Graham acknowledges the emotions and confusing responses people often feel when viewing the film. After the sobering viewing of *Birthday* the audience of young people is provided with some space, a critical distance from which to reflect, weigh and consider the implications of the events leading up to, and following the crash. The program themes, already outlined in Graham's introduction, are captured in the *Birthday* story as a cautionary tale. Foreshadowing disaster – *'As they say, all good things must come to an end!'* – the film depicts David and his friend at a crossroads. A decision, one action, can alter the path of many lives.

In *Birthday*, and 'Shannon' and 'Julie's' stories, the impact of peer pressure features prominently. In *Birthday* peer influence/pressure is depicted as a motivation to drive dangerously and irresponsibly, with the Friend reflecting: *'You know what's really sad about all of this, is that … it doesn't have to happen. I'll be just showing off in front of these guys'*. Responsibility is reinforced in the belated realisation that: *'Good mates are meant to look after their mates, aren't they?'* The issue of overtly risky behaviour, which becomes a focus of specific messages and promotion of behaviour and attitude change in the program, is signalled in the film, with the Friend admitting that he would be *'just taking a few risks on the road'*. It is an echo of the film-maker's own story. Shannon's friends, we are told, sped down the road and slammed into a bridge.

Consequences are starkly signposted. The obvious ones: loss of friends, students, daughters, sons. The narrator in *Birthday* is made aware of his friend David's presence in his life just as he is anticipating his looming absence. For the victim, a life cut short, the loss of a future and future potential: *'For as long as I can remember David he's always lived life to the fullest'*, the Friend tells the gathering, *'and in a couple of months he was going to live out his dream, and travel around the world'*. Complex feelings remain for those left behind. For Shannon, there is guilt mixed with relief that she hadn't succumbed to pressure to get in the car. For the school principals such as Jim and Graham, the strength of the feelings they experienced led to a choice to devote the remainder of their careers to road safety promotion. Some of the consequences for the narrator in *Birthday* include shame, guilt and social ostracism, all captured in his rueful observation: *'Well, I suppose I should really try and enjoy this moment because, no-one here is going to look at me in the same way again. Especially his parents'*.

We would like to take a moment here to reflect on the narrative structures at work in these stories. Certain features and strategies of narrative are key to the impact of these stories, particularly as they involve the play of time, and the idea of retrospective knowing. Eleanor Ochs and Lisa Capps (2001, p. 5) describe a standard narrative device that heightens dramatic effect, and emotional and moral engagement, in their study of 'foreshadowing' and 'backshadowing' in conversational narrative. Foreshadowing is where the story is constructed by the narrator in anticipation of known conclusions: 'the narrator knows what will follow and casts characters and events in terms of this future trajectory'. All the action in the 'Julie' story, for instance, is directed towards the central interest point of the crash at the end of the story. Additional information, such as the end of year break-up of school, her plans, serve to lend weight to the central task of the story.

Earlier we referred to the use of similar devices in the context of reflecting on the ways in which 'reflexive hindsight' enables the allegorical to work in Tim Winton's novel *Breath* (Kelly 2011). As a narrative technique 'hindsight provides us with a vantage point that we don't possess in the now, in the moments when we choose, embrace, stumble upon things that may be far reaching in consequence and significance – when we are young and/or old'. At-risk discourses expect young people to be able to develop 'prudential foresight' in order to 'imagine and colonise their futures in ways that can guard against damage, hurt, and pain' (Kelly 2011, p. 443).

Alongside this standard narrative technique, 'backshadowing' has a weightier moral and didactic role and impact. Backshadowing 'is a kind of retroactive foreshadowing in which the shared knowledge of the outcome of a series of events by narrator and listener is *used to judge the participant in those events as though they too should have known what was to come*' (Bernstein, quoted in Ochs and Capps 2001, p. 5). The example referenced by Ochs and Capps is the story of Jews in Austria in the 1930s, who are sometimes portrayed in narrative accounts as having seen the signs of encroaching Nazism without taking action to leave. The effect of backshadowing is to suggest that these Jews were naïve and somehow responsible for their fate.

The Fit to Drive stories, in common with stories told to teach the young across diverse human cultures, seek to develop an array of images, imagined experiences, algorithms for solving problems to guard against harm in the real world. Backshadowing is a recurring feature of the narrative momentum of these stories. In the Fit to Drive stories the audience knows that the outcome of each story will involve a fatal crash. They can identify the critical points at which the characters could adopt an alternative action that would avoid the outcome. For example, the young men in the overcrowded stolen car driven by an unlicensed driver could refuse to go along, and perhaps convince their friends as well, instead of getting involved in a nightmarish crash. The audience, depending on their perspective, may judge the characters as naïve, as irresponsible, as ignorant, or, simply unlucky. The Fit to Drive discourse casts them as unprepared, lacking knowledge, inexperienced, perhaps lacking decision-making and assertiveness skills. The story, and the way in which it is told, aims to lead the audience to an understanding of this perspective, with the accompanying realisation that different decisions and actions were/are required in such circumstances. This backshadowing is one of the significant techniques through which the audience gains insight and reflects on moral and practical choices. Backshadowing allows for the audience to develop the 'reflexive hindsight', the retroactive insight necessary to understand the question of 'right action' (Kelly 2011; Kamp and Kelly 2014).

The short film *Birthday* employs a backshadowing technique to powerful effect. The Friend, aware of the coming events, refers to his knowledge that later in the evening he will be responsible for his friend David's death in a car crash. The force of the backshadowing is augmented by the exuberance and laughter of the guests that greets references to the tragedy to come and the proud expressions from the young man's parents, as their ignorance persists in stark and disquieting contrast to the awareness of the best friend. The laughter and applause provide the backdrop to the stricken face of the Friend. The black humour in the film – with the presentation to David of a framed copy of his death certificate – is effectively used to increase the impact, the unexpected shock of the final words. In this instance the backshadowing effect is heightened by the foreknowledge of the main character, as well as that of the narrator/author and the audience. The character provides his own retrospective moral judgement in the midst of the narrative's forward momentum – as the action is occurring.

As Ochs and Capps (2001, p. 4) argue: 'All narrative exhibits tension between the desire to construct an over-arching storyline that ties together in a seamless explanatory framework and the desire to capture the complexities of the events experienced, including haphazard details, uncertainties, and conflicting sensibilities among protagonists.' Narratives, characterised by the compulsion to create 'a single line of development out of a multiplicity' in which 'alternatives once present disappear from view', are in danger of masking the complexities and ambiguities of 'reality'. In Fit to Drive there is a constant play with alternatives, but the alternatives are played out in the shadow stories, the eternal 'what ifs' of the individual tragedies. It is the 'what ifs' that remain in the frame. 'What if' the young people at the Monavale party had asked the parents to call another taxi? 'What if' the driver had made two trips? This is the premise of the TAC short film *Anything?*,[3] which involves a young man putting comic 'what if' scenarios to his best mate. In tests of loyalty and friendship his friend reluctantly agrees that he would take on some arduous challenges for his friend: play footy in steel wool underwear; run across Australia; consume a hundred hard boiled eggs. The humour turns sour when the shot pans to reveal the scene of a cemetery where the friends are sitting. The young man, who had evidently been injured, is speaking to his dead friend: 'Why did you let me speed?' The film asks the viewer to contemplate the alternative ending to the narrative, where the young man would have discouraged his friend from speeding.

'Sideshadowing', a related though less common narrative technique, stands in contrast, because of its ambiguity, to the relatively stable meaning systems of foreshadowing and backshadowing. Sideshadowing occurs when 'literary and historical narratives cast events as ambiguous, conflictual, unstable. Subject to constant revision, perhaps even unknowable' (Ochs and Capps 2001, p. 5). For literary critic Michael Bernstein (1994, p. 3) quoted in Ochs and Capps (2001, p. 6), 'sideshadowing stresses the significance of random, haphazard and inassimilable contingencies'. Rather than focussing on the 'power of a system to uncover an otherwise unfathomable truth', sideshadowing expresses the ever-changing nature of that truth and the absence of any predictive certainties in human affairs. This narrative perspective is recognised as allowing for deeper exploration and questioning of the story's subject. But it should also be acknowledged that: 'Nonlinear narration opens narration to multiple truths and perspectives and the realization that certain life experiences resist tidy, ready-at-hand interpretive frameworks' (Ochs and Capps 2001, p. 45). 'Sideshadowing' is not a storytelling technique that is at home in the Fit to Drive story world. Fit to Drive can find no place for such 'sideshadowing' and the ambiguities it raises. When it approaches dangerously close (as in the Monavale tragedy, with its pervasive sense of random forces at work) it leaves a sense of discomfort and dissatisfaction. Ambivalence and ambiguity must be made absent, manifestly or as Other. We will engage the limits and possibilities of this ambivalence later.

In the stories we have described here there is an unstable distinction between the 'fictional' (TAC film) and the historical/personal (Julie, Graham, Shannon). The historical/personal stories have their roots in the intensely personal stories of the people who have been instrumental in the development of the program. Many of those who become involved in Fit to Drive share the multiple burdens of a personal story about road trauma. Their story may have been, or become, part of the Fit to Drive story in their region, it may have been told in the workshop introduction, or it may be a privately felt and held burden. The narrative currents that flow through Fit to Drive – sometimes subterranean, sometimes visibly on the surface – have their source in the experience of individual people. The narratives that have become the 'official', sanctioned Fit to Drive stories have been fashioned, given acceptable, or manageable shape in their telling and retelling in these settings. Their telling in the staged ('theatrical') setting of the school based workshop diminishes their potential volatility, renders them 'safe' by circumscribing the content, and maintaining focus on the carefully managed message of this particular intervention. As the program has grown, and the number of presenters has increased (local area coordinator, MFB and police officers), attention has been paid to the careful scripting of the delivery of the MFB and police presentations. On occasion this has been ignored, even resisted, by some of the officers involved, who feel that their presentation would be made more effective, more affective, more 'real' by the telling of their own stories, or improvisation on the scripted stories. This has sometimes led to rambling accounts, dilution of the message and disruption of the story as learning strategy. At worst it has involved inappropriate, unprocessed, personal disclosure of experiences of loss and trauma.

The characteristics of story and narrative: lessons for health promotion

Up until this point we have been using both 'narrative' and 'story' in the descriptions of the introductory session. Story and narrative are terms that are often used interchangeably. Sometimes they are treated synonymously, and sometimes distinctions are made between the two. Many different definitions of narrative and story exist. In social research, psychology, anthropology and related theoretical fields, where the focus is on individual and social meaning making, and the way narrative gives form and meaning to lived experience, 'narrative' and 'story' are often used interchangeably. In everyday discourse each carries diverse meanings and both are used in many different contexts.

Even in literary studies it has been noted that it is not always meaningful or simple to distinguish between 'story' as a literary text and 'personal narrative' (Bakhtin 1981). In Fit to Drive there are representations of both personal narrative, and narrative which becomes a 'literary'/performance text. And, importantly, these narratives have evolved and been shaped over time to become 'sanctioned' stories that have a specific educational role and symbolic/cultural place in the Fit to Drive program and culture. For the purposes of this discussion and analysis we have taken 'narrative' to mean the process by which we order events and experience into a meaningful, 'tellable' order. Story, in this context, can be understood as a more or less formal, artfully constructed, medium that employs stylistic devices for aesthetic and meaningful effect.

For some, stories not only play a central role in the way we make sense of our lives, but constitute the means by which we construct our self-identity (Gergen and Gergen 1983). Donald E. Polkinghorne (1988, pp. 134–135) refers to the role of narrative in creating and organising our experience. He draws on the work of Paul Ricoeur to explore the place of narrative as 'the linguistically, hermeneutically reasoned expression of the human experience of time', noting that by 'telling stories and writing history, we provide a public shape for what ordinarily remains "chaotic, obscure, and mute"'. Life is 'lived above the objective plane and its instantaneous "nows"'. In this sense, 'Temporal existence draws the past and its possibilities into the present through tales and histories and it imaginatively anticipates the future consequences of activity by seeing them as reenactments of its repertoire of stories.'

Narrative 'is the cognitive structure that draws together temporal events into a coherent whole' (Polkinghorne 1991, p. 146). Polkinghorne's use of 'narrative' alludes to the *process* by which we render our lives and our experience meaningful and comprehensible. Other writers point to the way in which our sense of self and our social being are understood through the lens of story (Bruner 1990; McAdams 1996). Stories, from this perspective, are foundational to our understandings of our lives, our relationships, our ability to grasp concepts and ideas, the development of our moral sense:

> Narratives constantly grapple with forces of order and disorder, integrity and chaos, good and evil. We become much more aware of their presence here than in abstract formulations. This is clearly the reason why so many of the basic truths of world religions are presented in story form where they are so vividly portrayed and remembered.
>
> (Ellos 1994, p. 70)

Ochs and Capps (2001, p. 18) are, further, interested in identifying 'conversational narrative' as a distinctive form of narrative. Narrative, they maintain, is hard to pin down, it 'bows to no simple generic blueprint that sets it apart once and for all from other forms of discourse'. It does, however, have certain features that are common:

> Narrative is a cognitively and discursively complex genre that routinely contains some or all of the following discourse components: *description, chronology, evaluation*, and *explanation* ... Settings, for example, are built from *descriptions.* Classic plots depict both a linear or more complex

> *chronology* of unfolding events and an overarching *explanation* of why a particular event transpired at a particular point in the narrative sequence.

In their analysis of conversational narrative, Ochs and Capps (2001, p. 2) observe that personal narrative 'is a way of using language or another symbolic system to imbue life events with a temporal and logical order, to demystify them and establish coherence across past, present, and as yet unrealized experience'. This definition of narrative refers specifically to the organisation of events in a temporal, causal, sequence. The ordering of events is an important part of the attempt to create order in the midst of chaotic, messy, uncontrollable reality, giving sense, meaning or purpose to the cacophony of life which doesn't easily yield to meaning. Narrative is a means of constructing a sense of self and personal 'anchoring' in the world. Such a view introduces the idea that people consciously or unconsciously create and tell narratives to render coherent their experience, their 'selves'. Narrative activity (in conversation, 'ordinary social exchanges') is a way of 'developing frameworks for understanding events' (Ochs and Capps 2001, p. 2). Ochs and Capps reference Bakhtin's (1981) argument that all narrative requires two subjects, two 'consciousnesses' – an author/reader nexus. In Ochs and Capps' reading, it is the teller–interlocutor relationship which is crucial in shaping the narrative – the interlocutor helps construct the narrative. A situation that gives rise to the question: What is the place of 'internal-narratives'? A personal narrative may be internalised, but is nevertheless constructed with an internalised interlocutor. The narrator still tells and retells the story, in her mind, imagines an audience, constructs a sequence of events – a chronology – selects and 'detaches' the events, evaluates and takes a moral stance.

Although Ochs and Capps (2001, p. 2) are specifically interested in social/conversational narrative, the features they describe also apply to more formal narrative structures. Conversational narratives have the added dimension of interaction and dialogue, involving '*questions, clarifications, challenges*, and *speculations* about what might possibly have transpired'. Conversational narrative doesn't necessarily have the finished form of 'story'. 'Narrators have something to tell, but the details and the perspective are relatively inchoate; they are still in the middle of sorting out an experience'. Narratives are 'selections of reality' (Ochs and Capps 2001, p. 45), perspectives on events that express the 'moral stance' of the narrator, and which become 'real' in the telling.

In literature, narrative is associated with the 'voice' that tells the story. The narrator as distinct from the author. It involves the author's formal creation of 'narrator', with conscious, aesthetically determined choices. Personal narrative assumes the narrator is speaking for themselves. Ochs and Capps analyse a number of devices that are used in personal narrative. Personal narrative may involve a 'first telling' of the events and circumstances. Often, however, the speaker will have told the story many times. To themselves, as a stream of consciousness; to others as confidantes and casual interlocutors.

At some stage it becomes shared story. What is the relationship between story and narrative? Ochs and Capps (2001), though generally using narrative and story interchangeably, seem to regard 'story' as a more developed form of discourse, while narrative is imagined as being something more spontaneous and instinctive. Story appears as artful, finished text. The 'overarching storyline' is not necessarily present in narrative. Narrative, as the focus of their study, assumes the personal, meaning making function. They note literary critics' differentiation of literary and oral narratives – the former in finished state when we first begin to read/encounter it. Citing Langer (1991), they suggest that: 'oral testimony steers a less certain course, like a fragile craft veering through turbulent waters, unsure where a safe harbour lies – or whether one exists at all!' (Ochs and Capps 2001, p. 4).

'Story' most commonly overlaps with definitions of narrative when the focus is on the function of story as relating a sequence of events defined by a concern with, or interest in, 'what happened next?'. For Scheub (1998 p. 48), who is primarily interested in the various manifestations of story within specific African cultures, narrative simply provides the surface organisation for story. 'Narrative provides the story with a backbone', but 'the meaning of story has little to do with narrative, which has simple organizing functions to play'. For Scheub, story encompasses much more, however. Metaphor, image and emotion are woven together through the bare canvas of the narrative to compose 'story'.

In Fit to Drive the need for meaning and coherence – wresting back order from the chaos of road trauma – for both individuals and community, finds its outlet in story. In constructing the repertoire of Fit to Drive stories, in ordering events into a chronological sequence, there is a promise that a certain level of understanding can be gained, that it is possible to achieve a fleeting sense of control. By tidying these events into a series of cause and effect relations (*risks*) it is possible to *think forward*, to project to *future events* and restructure the events into something that is within one's grasp and controllable. Yet, this process of 'colonising the future' (Giddens 1991) highlights the tension in the very character of story. On the level of individual narrative it is a means to gain control, coherence, meaning. On the other hand, for the audience, its power lies in the satisfaction of the drama itself, which may not depend on the neat resolution and coherence of events.

Hayden White (1980, p.27) cautions that the 'value attached to narrativity in the representation of real events ... arises out of a desire to have real events display the coherence, integrity, fullness and closure of an image of life that can only be imaginary'. It is reasonable that, for those in Fit to Drive who have been 'touched by the toll', these 'goods' – coherence, integrity, fullness – will be sought after, strived for. In grief, people search for meaning, reasons, coherence and closure. Can the randomness and terror of a young person's death in a car crash be rendered bearable by being turned into story? This act of 'sense-making' from *no-sense* – constructing a narrative – carries the hope of wresting back order and intelligibility even as we are cautioned that: 'Story provides insight, but never closure' (Scheub 1998, p. 3).

For some analyses of narrative fiction, narration equals the *telling* of the story – the process of production, the organisation of the telling: 'Unless it is told a story would not be a narrative, and without being narrated or written it would not be a text' (Rimmon-Kenan 1983, p. 4, quoted in Scheub 1998, p. 297). The narrative text is 'defined by the story (its "object") and the narration (the process of its production)'. Generally, however, these distinctions appear to be more relevant to literary studies, where there is a concern to differentiate between story (narrative) and *narration* – the art of writing and speaking (though these can become confused). In the end, for Scheub (1998, p. 51), narrative is:

> chiefly an organising device that holds image in linear embrace, with its single-minded concern for the movement from conflict to resolution. It is the cerebral part of the story, being the repository of obvious ideas and homilies, and in its deceptively quiet nature it seldom betrays the cauldron of emotions seething beneath its surface.

For Scheub (1998, p. 47), then, story is greater than a sequence of events: 'Story is the totality of activities that comprise storytelling performance, each of which is a crucial ingredient. Narrative is not the crucial activity as far as the eventual experience of story is concerned'. Whether construed as a fundamental organising function of the human mind, or a linguistic and cultural 'tool', narrative and story are fused into the one mode of discourse, whereby both narrative and story represent the organisation of events into sequences that cohere, in various ways, to make meaning. For Scheub what distinguishes story from narrative is the rich panoply of image, rhythmic movement, evocative metaphor and abundant storehouse of emotion to be found on and beneath its surfaces. Emotion has the core task of 'binding' the story, which incorporates image, narrative, rhythm, trope (metaphor), patterning (and performance).

In our analysis of the Fit to Drive workshop 'narrative' is used to describe two interrelated concepts. It is both the process by which people construct personal understanding of experience by ordering and arranging events and experience into (linear) order, and the larger, organising schema related to Fit to Drive's presentation and explanation of the complexities of young people, road use and crashes. This incorporates the general assemblage of stories (which involve 'narration'), selected information and interpretations, as well as modes of engagement, that constitute the Fit to Drive workshop 'model'. In this context stories structure the narrative that gives shape and purpose to Fit to Drive workshops. Each of the stories could be told elsewhere to structure a different narrative, but here they give the Fit to Drive workshop a particular shape, they serve a particular purpose.

Narrative is present in Fit to Drive – not only as the grand narrative of the Fit to Drive sanctioned stories and message, whether viewed as tragedy or morality tales (both are present) – but also in the power of personal narrative. Young people and facilitators in conversations that emerge in spaces opened by these stories employ the form of conversational narrative. The emotional, conceptual shift when we add 'personal' – 'personal narrative' – to the consideration of narrative is interesting. It reflects an internal world, at once authoritative and legitimate, and at the same time marginalised and provisional, because it is 'subjective'.

Story, empathy and understanding

Kerry's story: understanding Jim

I first met Jim and heard his story when we did some training in the west, at Victoria University (VU). He had organised the funding of Fit to Drive in some schools, and had worked hard at building up links with VU departments (Education mainly, but also some links with Youth Work) and recruited around twenty students to be trained. I had heard about him and his work from Graham and Bern. He came along to the first day of training, bringing boxes of showbags, pamphlets, stickers, drink bottles (police 'Look Bike' campaign) for the participants. Modest in demeanour, Jim didn't seek to promote himself in any way, or to take a prominent place in the 'public face' of the program. However, being a political animal seems to be part of the role of a secondary school principal, and he was extremely good at mobilising resources as well as support for the program. On this occasion we asked him to say a few words of welcome to the new group of facilitators (in-training). As part of his welcome he spoke of his own background and told the story of his young students who had lost their lives in road crashes, and how one of these stories had found its way into the TAC film, made by one of the student's friends, that was about to be shown to the group. Telling the story, and recalling his own devastation during that period, Jim became visibly upset, a reaction that I would witness a number of times, with different people, over the years. Jim, in telling that story, returns to the feelings, bodily sensations, perceptions, images that accompanied, were an integral part of, that experience. His are embodied memories. Graham reflects on the fact that he tells (must tell) 'Julie's Story' anew each time. He describes it as a new experience each time he recounts it. Why? It is, in some crucial way, an 'embodied experience'.

Over numerous training sessions there have been facilitators who have shared, or referred to (without dwelling on it) their own loss of friends or relatives, as a result of car crashes. Without delving into the circumstances (training was not the appropriate place to do this) it has been obvious that the personal narratives of many of these people have included powerfully felt stories relating to road trauma. People entering 'helping' professions are expected, as part of reflective practice, to have 'worked through' personal issues and past experiences that may continue to impact on their engagement, judgement and 'professional distance'. People who are motivated by their experience with road trauma, but who may not necessarily be adequately equipped to play a positive educative or activist role, can become a problem in road safety. If this arises in Fit to Drive it becomes a sensitive issue that needs to be managed and dealt with appropriately.

People have noted, and been drawn toward, the particular spirit – the 'heart' that distinguishes Fit to Drive as a school and community program. It is this intense engagement of many of those involved, and the respect accorded their experience, which spills over to the entire program (personnel) and – importantly – is combined with the professional orientation and practice (avoiding populist, reactive responses; awareness of need for professional judgement and distance, etc.) which contributes to, builds and defines the nature of Fit to Drive. In this sense we can imagine, as Spinosa et al. (1997) did in a study of Mothers Against Drink Driving (MADD), the formation of a 'community of interest'. The Fit to Drive 'community of interest' has shared stories, and recognises and respects the power of those stories, just as their 'tellers' reflect on and respect the fact that they are using, drawing upon the tragic stories of others for the purpose of education.

Les Todres (2007, p. 3), reflecting on the nature of understanding from a phenomenological perspective, notes that: 'phenomenology grounds human enquiry in a way that marries 'head' and 'heart''. The acceptance of 'heart' – the involvement of the emotions, and the bodily awareness that entails – as a vital component of understanding echoes the emphasis on emotion as key to story and as an integral element of Fit to Drive. It is this combination of 'head and heart' that is the key to this 'community of interest' – the prominence allowed the 'heart' in the message/story of the program. And it is the balance of the two that is the foundation for the educational philosophy of the program, which strives to achieve a deep engagement, awareness and understanding in its target audience by, first of all, engendering a connection with the experience of the subjects of the various stories.

What does it mean: to *comprehend* a human experience? Todres (2007, p. 10), in discussing this question draws upon Dilthey's term *nacherleben* – to 're-enact', according to Todres' translation (it may also be understood/translated as 're-experience'): 'Within this perspective, to comprehend a human experience, whether one's own or that of another, is to bring it into the light of one's own possibilities – and thus to re-enact it.'

In Fit to Drive individual stories are interwoven, contributing/offering different moments – of insight, revelation, instruction, empathy. Layered between are the stories of each new participant – young people, teachers, observers, new facilitators – told and untold. The stories that are told emerge in the workshop discussions. There's not always time to share these with the whole group, but students share them amongst themselves. Other – often snatches of – stories are told in the large group: *'When we were driving in the Northern Territory …', 'My brother and his mates were driving up in Craigieburn when …', 'A friend of mine was in a crash last Christmas and …'*

The workshop invites students to engage on a level of empathy – to 're-enact', re-experience, the stories and experiences of others as told in the workshop, and to enfold them into their own being. The stories that are communicated evoke empathy and participation. In doing so, there is a need to overcome deeply entrenched mistrust of 'emotion' or 'emotive arguments'. A mistrust of the emotional that we will return to later.

The stories that are *untold* in the workshop, the stories that are both manifestly absent and absent as Other, provide other dimensions to the meaning making that occurs in the workshops. These stories form part of each young person's individual history and create the ground on which 'the seeds are scattered and bear fruit' (to use an analogy often employed by youth workers and health educators). These stories are manifestly absent. They are imagined as being there, as forming a significant part of the Fit to Drive hinterland. Graham has often argued that each young person who comes to a Fit to Drive workshop enters that space as a stage/wayside stop along their personal journey, and each one brings their own journey experience – and stories – with them. The stories they encounter in Fit to Drive connect with, and spark off, their own stories and characters, and engage and entangle with their own experiences, feelings and thoughts.

Todres (2007, p. 15), citing Husserl, conceptualises understanding as a movement that proceeds from a 'home' towards the 'other': 'It can be meaningful to talk of understanding as a journey of appropriation and transgression – an interplay between the familiar and unfamiliar'. Fit to Drive, in terms of the goods that it seeks to produce, provides a relatively safe space in which to play out the journey from 'home' – the world of familiar understanding and knowledges – to explore and experience new ideas, concepts and stories, and integrate these into a new understanding: 'For Husserl, to understand is to imagine, to transgress the concrete event and enter the horizon of the world, and to find its unities for back home' (Todres 2007, p. 16). Playing with the idea of understanding as emanating from a self within 'home', venturing towards the 'out there-ness' of 'other', understanding is conceived as 'bridge-making'. New perspectives offered by the 'out-there' enrich and illuminate 'home'. 'Home is transformed and adventures become meaningful for home. Understanding is bridgemaking … a mixing of interpenetrating worlds' (Todres 2007, p. 16).

In this view, it is the new perspectives and experiences offered by the Fit to Drive encounter, which lead to new understanding. These new perspectives and experiences require young people to journey from their 'home', and to be transformed by the experience, the 'adventure'. The stories in Fit to Drive are effective because they are affective. But they only become transformative (in the sense of young people becoming *fit to drive*) when young people can rewrite and re-enact the story. For example, the final participatory learning activity at the end of the workshop involves the students reading a scenario, to produce and role play (enact) the collectively generated solutions leading to positive endings (outcomes). In formulating, conducting, reviewing and evaluating this strategy for meaning making, great emphasis is placed on providing openings, opportunities for practising the skills, using the language and demeanour of assertive, self-protective behaviours, to 'rewrite' the scene.

Narrative quest and the pursuit of the moral in health promotion

William Ellos (1994, p. 66), referencing the work of Roland Barthes, suggests that the 'mythic' involves 'entering into a world of sharing and shared values', and that the mythic, in this sense, is central to processes of interpretation and the construction of (shared) meaning. The story of the 'beginnings' of Fit to Drive, with their foundations in tragedy, has a primal resonance, with overtones of the passing on of mythic stories. It is the foundation of community by means of communal stories. Ellos' interpretation of the place of myth, as a particular form of narrative, in the construction of meaning offers a means by which we may understand the central place accorded to values in Fit to Drive. The program's ethos and educational philosophy is firmly based on the idea that the exploration, acknowledgement and questioning of values is the key to people's integration of (new) knowledge and behavioural intentions. The small group activities are designed specifically to generate opportunities to explore values in group discussion.

In Fit to Drive the ground for this discovery of values is laid in the scene-setting stories. These constitute the store of myth guarded by the program. The mythic dimension of the program incorporates meaning-laden narrative, but also recognisable archetypes. For example, the tragic figure at the centre of 'Julie's Story' is, we are told, the 'popular girl'. The storytellers know how to draw together the elements of a powerful story, though not wanting to play into stereotypes: 'Not that this is relevant, but …' When presenters commence the workshop with a retelling of 'Julie's Story', they build at the same time the story of the beginnings of Fit to Drive. The story, in its generational 'move' from its origins has become history/myth. The gathering of school principals to confront the problem has the weight, the resonance, of a 'council of war', responding to a threat (with sometimes problematic resonances with other 'wars' on modern targets – the global 'war on drugs', or the 'war on terror').

The philosopher Alasdair MacIntyre (1981, p. 122) ties in the human need to explore and discover the answers to fundamental questions of moral life with the idea of the 'narrative quest' – 'the pursuit of goodness in the course of narration'. Ochs and Capps (2001, p. 50) draw on MacIntyre's concept of narrative quest to explore the central place of narrative in the pursuit of the moral life. Narratives not only express social, cultural and personal world views, but are the instrumental means of building moral meaning, not only in audience/interlocutor, but the narrator herself: 'Everyday narration of life experience is a primary medium for moral education, in that each recounting involves piecing together the moral meaning of events' (ibid.). This interpretation recognises the 'moral stance' of a narrative as fluid and uncertain, subject to change, within the receiving and within the telling. The telling of a narrative with an intended moral message is dependent on the capacity and preparedness of the audience to make a shift in their understanding. But the narrative act may also involve a challenge to the moral stance of the teller. The audience response, the perceived response, may constitute such a challenge. For Ochs and Capps (2001, p. 18), a narrative is imbued from its inception with a moral and aesthetic '*evaluation* of actions, emotions, thoughts, and worldly conditions'. A moral position, a moral stance lies at the core, and is fundamental to the understanding, of narrative: 'Central to narrative perspective is the *moral stance* assumed by tellers and protagonists. Rooted in community and tradition, moral stance is a disposition towards what is good or valuable and how one ought to live in the world' (Ochs and Capps 2001, p. 45). A moral stance, whether in conversational, or more formal, narrative forms, may be presented as certain and constant, or expressed as uncertain and fluid (Ochs and Capps 2001, p. 20).

The Fit to Drive workshop, in ways that are similar to many school based health promotion interventions, provides a space in which young people are invited to reflect on, and share, their experience, and in effect develop, articulate and adopt a moral stance. This is partially achieved through the unfolding of personal narratives. The students in the workshop are encouraged to articulate their own (moral) position towards certain dilemmas and situations presented to them. In the process of expressing their views they frequently construct their argument with reference to examples that they draw from life experience – their own, or someone else's. In the 'Values clarification' activity, as the students huddle in groups to share their reasons for adopting an 'agree' or 'disagree' position on various statements, young people will often articulate their opinions in the context of narrating a personal story, or the story of a friend, sibling or parent. The very process of narrating the events or circumstances engenders a questioning, clarifying, rethinking: a destabilising effect that may call their viewpoint (moral stance) into question.

Road safety education, at first glance prosaic, associated as it is with the essentially practical and mundane concerns of road rules, speed limits, alcohol and other drug restrictions, offers a productive space in which to explore complex moral concerns. In this it is similar to other areas of moral education, such as sexual health, or alcohol and other drug education, all of which impart factual knowledge in the context of the exploration of values, attitudes and ethics (Carmody 2009). In Fit to Drive these moral concerns, central to the educational focus of the program, are most vividly captured in story. Fit to Drive may be seen, in one sense, as a cycle of stories: different stories recapitulating elemental themes and moral questions and dilemmas build upon each other to become something more than the sum of the individual stories alone. The core elements comprising the individual stories build the narrative momentum of the workshop. Stories give shape to the moral vision and message of the program.

Stories have been a major generative force behind the 'discovery' of the problem of young people and road crashes, both within public policy, and more specifically in the establishment and growth of the Fit to Drive program. These stories are present as a major moral force and source of understanding – an integral conduit into the emotional connection with the problem. An awareness of the power of stories has meant that within Fit to Drive stories are carefully circumscribed and managed. This caution is extended to the management of personal stories shared within the small groups by both young people and facilitators.

MacIntyre's idea of the 'narrative quest' resonates with the image of 'journey', which is often invoked by Fit to Drive members who have a long history with the program and young driver safety. Both Graham and Jim, in telling their story, use the metaphor of *journey* to describe their experiences, from the experience of being thrown into dealing with their grief-stricken school communities, to the reorientation of their professional (and to a degree) personal lives towards road safety, and young drivers in particular: 'So, that was my journey – the journey's been very significant.' The journey is an archetypal metaphor and narrative device, characteristic of the epic, and immediately arouses associations with elements we link with the epic: personal epiphany or challenge; enlightenment; forward movement through difficulties. In describing the process that communities go through in their search for solutions to young driver crashes, Graham also repeatedly refers to journey, in the context of his own self-discovery; the community's 'journey' beyond grief to understanding and action; to young people's 'journey' in the development of life experience, knowledge and moral development. Jim's journey involved the realisation that: 'I needed maybe to do something about this.' Jim's self-described 'journey' is, in this sense, a 'narrative quest':

> It is in the course of the quest and only through encountering and coping with the various particular harms, dangers, temptations, and distractions which provide any quest with its episodes and incidents that the goal of the quest is finally to be understood. A quest is always an education both as to the character of that which is sought and in self-knowledge.
>
> (MacIntyre 1981, p. 219)

An aside: The 'road movie' (for example, *Thelma and Louise, Easy Rider, Little Miss Sunshine*), as a late twentieth-century cultural artefact and archetype, gives a central place to the motor car, as machine and trope, for 'driving', literally and figuratively, the journey, through time and space, through personal transformation. The road movie, and the cultural tropes it plays with, and puts into play, is another absence (as Other) in/from Fit to Drive. It sits, unacknowledged, in the hinterlands that give Fit to Drive, as a school based health promotion intervention for young people, its structure and purpose.

The challenges and opportunities here are many and complex. We have shown that they are potentially productive in exploring the emotional, the affective and the aesthetic dimensions of story, and of meaning making in school based health promotion. In the midst of all the messiness, complexity, ambiguity and ambivalence that characterises our lives, stories work to give meaning, purpose and structure to our lives. In framing, making and telling stories – to ourselves, to our interlocutors – the devices we deploy, the choices we make, the things that we make present, or manifestly absent, or absent as Other, are implicated in the struggle to make and communicate meaning. The meanings we make, that we communicate, are unstable, open to interpretation, up for grabs, always characterised by ambivalence and ambiguity. Even if we plan, in the making and the telling, to minimise ambiguity and misunderstanding – 'Let's be clear …' – we can never be unambiguously clear. The parts of the whole are unstable. The sum of the parts is unstable.

Earlier, we noted the difficulties that ambivalence, ambiguity and instability create for school based health promotion programs such as Fit to Drive, and the need to frame a program with clear, achievable ends in mind. We noted the 'goods' that we aim to produce; the 'right' forms of thinking that we want young people to develop and deploy; the forms of agency that we want them to enact (more on this later). All of these have in mind, and emerge from the framing of, narratives that promise to impose some order, reason and meaning on the unruliness and disorder of the world: the unruliness and disorder of bodies, minds and souls. As we have already suggested, school based health promotion seeks to do these things in the particular *irreality* that makes schools more or less governable spaces (Rose 1999). This necessarily limited, constrained space of possibilities enables certain things to be thought, said and done (reason, risk, rationality), has a lot of trouble with allowing other things to be thought, said and done (aesthetics, emotions, un-reason, ambivalence, complexity), and just cannot allow other things to be thought, said and done (erotics, pleasure).

In the ways that we have been talking about the things able to be thought, said and done, schools, and the health promotion interventions that are allowed in schools, make certain things present, certain things manifestly absent, and certain things absent as Other. It is in the stories that are told in these irreal spaces that the unstable, shifting, complex and ambivalent relations between presence, manifest absence and absence as Otherness becomes, at least momentarily, clear. In making these presences and absences clear we can ask of ourselves, and others, are these the sorts of stories that we want to tell? Are there better stories? Even, in examining the stories we currently tell, in framing the 'goods' we currently seek to produce, are there, indeed, other 'goods' we have not even imagined before? Other stories that haven't been told, that could be told?

Notes

1 Burton Secondary College, June 2009: introductory session.
2 This film was produced under the TAC's 'Make a Film Make a Difference' program. This was a competition for young people under twenty-five, who were invited to write a short film proposal on a road safety theme. The winning entrants were given funding and support to develop their idea into a short film, which then received public distribution through TAC.
3 Shown in the final, plenary, session of the workshop.

6 A Greek tragedy

Chaos and control

The Monavale tragedy

November 2009. At Brandon Glen Secondary College, a school in a working-class, ethnically diverse suburb about ten kilometres north of Melbourne, 'Shane', the MFB officer, is presenting the Monavale case study.

'So, now I'm going to create a picture in your minds, of the scene I'm about to set. How I would like you to do that is, to put your head down, close your eyes for a moment, and picture this situation, alright?' He waits until all the students have closed their eyes. 'There's a big country house outside the suburban area of Sydney – picture somewhere like Kinglake. Does anyone know where Kinglake is? Yeah, in the mountains. That's right, so, eighty young eighteen-year-olds have gone there for a birthday party. About thirty or forty of them are boys from a private boys' school, and the other half are girls from a neighbouring girls' private school. The parents of one of the people own this home, and they've made it available on this weekend for a birthday party. Some of the people who've got their licence have driven there. Some have got a lift with others, and some people have got there by taxi. The party's gone really well, everyone's had a good time. The parents who own the place have done all the right things to make sure everything is going well. It's now about one o'clock in the morning, and people are heading off for home. Again, the parents have done the right thing. They've organised a whole team of taxis to come out and pick up the people who needed a lift. They see that all of that is in place, and the parents go off to bed. But there are eight people – two groups of four, who are yet to leave. And it's those eight people that we're now going to focus on. So, that's the picture – ok? Hold that picture in your head that you've created, because we're now going to play it out here.

'I need a few volunteers. Girls, can I have six of you from along here (to the front row), just step out the front. It's not a speaking part, OK? One, two, three, four, two more – girls? And two guys on the end of the row here, you two, could you come down here?' The students follow Shane, who directs them, 'Can you just come around the back here for a moment?' Shane is calmly shepherding the students to stand at the back of the group of chairs, which he has gathered into a shape at the front of the auditorium. 'OK, we have two groups of four here.

We have this group, with –' He approaches a student, and, peering at her name tag, says, 'Jess – who is the owner of this beautiful Volkswagen hatchback.' (laughter as Shane points out the white plastic chairs representing the car) 'A lovely car,' smiles Shane. 'This is the hatch at the back, and as you can see it's a four seater car. Jess owns this car, and she's very proud of her car, but, Jess is not driving this car home tonight, because Jess knew that she'd be having a few drinks at the party. And the group appointed Emily as their designated driver to drive them home. It's one o'clock in the morning, they're about to pile into the car to drive home, Emily's about to hop into the driver's seat, when all of a sudden Anita says, "Hang on a minute, Emily, you're the designated driver, but I saw you have a few drinks during the night. You're not allowed to drive, as we've just heard in the police presentation. You're going to be over zero." [1] *'Anita –' Shane goes to stand next to her, '– is a champion netball player' (laughter) 'and Anita has a big match tomorrow, so hasn't had a drink all night. Had a good time, but hasn't had a drink. So Anita says to the other girls, "I'll drive." So the girls hop in the car, with Anita in the driver's seat.' Shane invites Anita to take her seat in the 'car'. As she hesitates, Shane asks, 'You know where to sit?' Laughter, and Anita good naturedly sits in the 'car'.*

'Hop in, girls,' says Shane, and the girls quickly move to take up positions. Shane continues: 'And, everything looks fine, and they're about to head off, when all of a sudden Jess spots four young people who have missed out on a taxi. The parents have missed one group when they ordered the taxis, and these guys have got no way of getting home. Those taxis won't come back, because it's way out in the country and it's late at night. And all the other cars with spare seats in them have gone. Jess turns to this group and very kindly says, "I'll give you a lift, pile in," and they do.'

Shane turns towards the audience and invites two boys and two girls to join the group in the 'car'. Laughter, as one of the boys immediately rushes to get in the car. Shane waylays him and directs him to the back. 'In the back, boys in the back. Girls, in the back seat!' The girls laughingly sit on the knees of the students already in the 'back seat'. Shane goes around to the boys, who are sitting, face outwards in the seats representing the 'hatch' He gently pushes their heads down, squashing them in the space. 'You have to remember this is a hatchback, and –' (he goes around the 'car', gently pushing the girls in) '– you have to be able to close the doors.' Another little nudge. Laughter, and Shane goes to the front to address the audience from there. 'Now, remember', he says, looking at the audience, 'Anita has volunteered to be the driver of this car, because of the situation I described before. She's now got a little bit more on her plate. She's now dealing with seven people who are, as you can see, wildly excited because they've been at the party.' Like a conductor, Shane orchestrates their acting: 'Wildly excited!' he enthuses, waving his arms. 'Having a great time!' He points at the students in the 'car', who are enthusiastically miming their excitement. 'They've all been drinking, texting each other on the phone while they're in the car, all that sort of thing. One o'clock in the morning. Anita has never driven this car before, and it's just started to rain outside. Anita turns to Jess – remember, the owner of the car – and says to Jess: "Too many people in the car." Jess says, "Not a problem Anita, I've done it before, and it's not a problem." In fact, Jess was actually going to volunteer to ride in the hatch, which I'm having trouble – (he gently kicks the boys' feet back in the 'hatch' space) – closing. But, these two guys are actually keen on a couple of the girls in the car' (laughter, grins exchanged between the boys) 'and they've volunteered that they'll ride in the hatch.

'OK,' Shane says, moving back to the front. 'Here's the scene. Late at night, overloaded car, people drinking – not the driver, but the others. It's raining outside now. Anita's never driven this car before. How many tennis balls have we got going around now?' Some answers come from the audience: 'Heaps.' 'Think of that workshop this morning,' Shane reminds the group.[2]

'OK, you've got the picture, and I want to say thank you to the volunteers, you can go back now.' There are enthusiastic cheers, and claps as the students return to their seats. 'And if we could have just left it at that, that would be fine. But unfortunately that is a true story. And I'm now going to show you how the rest of that story plays out.'

Our attention is directed to the screen, as a film appears, commencing with the MFB and CFA logos. Fit to Drive Road Crash Case Study *announces the title shot. A female newsreader appears, talking earnestly to the screen.*

'In a country where the car is king,' she intones, 'getting your driver's licence becomes a rite of passage. But, too often that new-found freedom turns to tragedy. A third of all road fatalities involve drivers who are under 25.'

The scene shifts to footage of a car driving at night. The image opens with the bright lights of an oncoming car piercing the vision of the driver, from whose perspective we are viewing the scene. The road looms into our vision in front of us, as the car travels along the dark road, between the illuminated road markers. It feels claustrophobic, unsafe. A female voiceover commentates: 'As a learner you are driving at the safest period of driving – you're at your lowest risk. Then you change to your probationary or provisional licence where the first six months is the highest risk period that you face as a driver.' As her voice fades out a soundtrack of ominous music encroaches. A male voice speaks: 'It's the time of life when you're most inexperienced as a driver, often there's alcohol involved, and often at that time of life there's a lot of peer passengers involved as well, so there's that greater element of distraction. Those combined certainly contribute to a heightened risk.'

The voice continues with the litany of risk as the footage on the screen turns into a night-time scene of a car crash, a scene of devastation, wet night, a small car, buckled and bent into a crumpled pile of metal. Discordant sounds of violins and other stringed instruments crescendo into an urgent soundtrack. We can now see a number of cars – two? three? – the desolate sight of crash wreckage, a yellow-coated fire officer picking his way around the debris, emergency vehicles. A new voice in the background, as we see shots of crash sites – poles, trees, with the familiar flower tributes placed around them. The voice belongs to a doctor, whom we see in head shot, recognisable by his stethoscope and, as the shot pans out, by the equipment and surroundings that denote a hospital setting, describing the frustration of dealing with crash casualties. 'Working with this, day to day, it gets frustrating.'

A new title appears on the screen: 'Crash study', with newspaper photos of a car wreck, school photos of two smiling young men, with the headline 'Schoolboys killed'. A young man's voice is heard over the images: 'I've been in the boot of a car before. You need to get somewhere, so you all pile in. I think, yes, it's about the driver taking responsibility in that sort of situation, because ...'

The image turns to a television news report, showing the crash scene. The female reporter is explaining: 'The VW Golf had no less than eight teenagers when the car lost control and slid back first into a telegraph pole. [The boys] were riding in the boot. They died of massive injuries.' (photos of the boys in a football team group shot appear on the screen). 'Today the driver, who cannot be identified because she was seventeen at the time, faced a committal hearing on two counts of dangerous driving, and driving causing death. She was chauffeuring a group home after a party in April last year when the crash happened.' There is footage of the young woman, face blurred to prevent identification, arriving at court with her lawyers and family. The news reporter continues: 'In court she repeatedly broke down into sobs. The owner of the car, the daughter of a well-known businessman,' (images of the car owner) 'told the court she'd often driven the car with boys in the boot before, insisting there was never a problem with it. In fact on the night, she intended to ride in the boot herself, but the boys insisted the girls take a seat inside the car. At the heart of the defence case was that there was nothing wrong with the way the car was driven, lawyers arguing the driver was not speeding or driving recklessly, and that there was no trace of alcohol in her system. The prosecution said that the fact she had so many people on board, and she was behind the wheel of a car she'd never driven before, at one o'clock in the morning, and in rainy conditions, was enough. The hearing's expected to run for three days.'

The commentary and images fade, and against the shadowy background of the boys' photos, the words silently appear in succession:

Peer pressure … Responsibility … Impacts … Choices

Shane's voice breaks the silence of the room. 'First of all, a few details about that film. You will have noticed that the driver was seventeen. It happened in New South Wales, where you can get your licence at seventeen. So, she was a licensed driver. But, because she was seventeen, because she was under eighteen, the law legally treats her as a minor. That's why she couldn't be identified on screen.

'A few things about that situation: that driver was licensed, hadn't been drinking, was trying to do all the right things, but, was clearly driving an overloaded car. When you break into workshops we're going to be analysing that situation in terms of those four terms that came up at the end.

'Let me talk briefly about some of the impacts that followed straight after that situation. That girl was an outstanding year twelve student, would have

gone on to university – would have got straight A's in her subjects. After that crash she missed forty-four days of school. Ended up not sitting for her year 12 exams, didn't complete her year 12. Twelve months later she was picked up on a drink driving charge. And a short while after that she was charged again, with substance abuse-related charges. She became ostracised by the others in her group, in other words isolated from her peers. In fact, some of the people in that car testified against her in that court case. She was in fact found not guilty in that court case, but you can see that, clearly, it affected the rest of her life. One of the ambulance drivers who attended that scene hasn't worked again to this day, due to the trauma of that crash.

'We're now going to break up into groups and analyse that scenario.'

Following the police presentation the focus of the workshop is centred on the Metropolitan Fire Brigade's (MFB) presentation of the 'Monavale' case study. As we have seen, the case study examines the circumstances of the crash and the reverberations that ricocheted through peer groups and communities, and irrevocably changed individual lives. It was developed as an educational program for senior secondary students, involving both video and group discussion activities.

The case study depicts a complex and dramatic story that forms the basis for an extended group discussion session in the workshop. It re/presents a difficult moral tableau that serves to stimulate thinking and debate about responsibility and 'right action' in which each character in the scenario has a moral decision to make, and each workshop participant has to consider that decision in the light of the information that is available to them. Students work in groups to tease out the issues under the headings of 'choice', 'peer pressure', 'responsibility' and 'impacts', exploring the motivations and responsibility of the various characters, the decisions that led to the sequences of events, and the consequences arising from the crash. The subheadings reflect the key workshop themes: factors that are seen to put young people at risk, in this case 'peers'; values ('responsibility'); the future-oriented focus of risk as an expression of (negative) possibilities ('impacts'); and the idea of young people as choosing agents ('choice'). Sometimes the students break up into groups in the large space, and the MFB officers, with support from the facilitators, workshop the case study. Sometimes the group work for this segment is conducted in the second small group workshop.

This chapter explores certain dimensions of road safety risk as representing, in significant ways, long-standing questions of the struggle between Fate and Reason, the capacity and uses of rationality to impose order from chaos, to assert control in a sea of randomness. We examine the ways in which many of the stories that are told or emerge from health promotion interventions resonate with the deeply embedded Western literary traditions of *the tragic*. Stories such as Monavale exemplify the distinctive features of tragedy, as first established by Aristotle in ancient Greece and developed in later European traditions of dramatists such as Shakespeare and Schiller. Central to the dynamic of tragedy is the interplay of Fate, of individual character, and the influences of the competing, and complementary, life forces: celebratory, wild Dionysian, and measured, restrained Apollonian. We want to develop and extend an argument that certain dimensions of young people's health related risks represent, in significant ways, long-standing questions of the struggle between Fate and Reason, and the capacity and uses of rationality to impose order from chaos, to assert control in a sea of randomness.

Kerry's story: Aeschylus or Aesop?

October 2009, MFB Training Centre

Graham and I are observing a training session for MFB officers who are preparing to become Fit to Drive presenters. The trainers recreate the activity as it is presented in the school workshops, with today's participants undertaking the same learning process as the year 11 students, followed by a discussion in relation to their role as presenters.

John sets the scene, arranging seven seats at the front of the room to represent the car, getting participants to adopt the places of the young people in the car. He explains how the young woman had reluctantly become recruited to drive after the designated driver, as well as car owner, had been drinking alcohol; how the numbers of young people wanting a lift grew beyond the capacity of the car; how two young men jump into the boot and two young women were sitting on the knees of other passengers. The group is told how the driver mouths: 'Too many people.' The group joke around noisily in the car, as it would have occurred, and John throws in some tennis balls, to represent the distractions for the driver. John asks: 'What now?', and runs the film that shows the news reports that follow the story. The overloaded car, as we know, goes out of control and crashes on the wet road, and the two young men are killed. The news report focuses on the court case. The young woman, we hear, is charged with culpable driving.

The story always upsets me. What troubles me is the way those involved turn against the young driver, who was only seventeen at the time. They blame and ostracise her, although the judge acquits her of the dangerous driving charges, and names all those involved equally responsible. I recoil at the way the 'friends' and their parents (though not all), turn on the young woman. I respond viscerally to the image of the young woman car owner, who is shown walking from the court, apparently nonchalantly picking food from a take-away paper bag, her father's arm protectively guiding her from the court. In contrast, it seems to me, to the fragile demeanour of the driver, her parents also protective, but appearing more vulnerable. Is this my imagination? Am I projecting my sympathy on them? This, quite likely, is partly a product of the way the image and commentary has been framed by the news: 'her [the car-owner's] father, a successful businessman'. I imagine the driver's family, their tragedy overshadowing the pitifully sad story of the two dead boys. An additional dimension: their parents – they are country people, and the boys' death has devastated the town – are anxious, we are told, to exonerate the young driver from blame. Totally entering the world of the story, I react with abhorrence to the pack, vigilante mentality of the friends and their families who have turned on the girl. She, we learn later, suffering emotional distress, has to repeat year 12, because she missed so much school. Formerly a keen sportswoman, a year after the crash she was picked up on drink-driving offences, and was reported to be suffering from depression.

For the first time, having seen this together many times, I express my reactions to Graham, and find an immediate affirmation and sympathy with my feelings. We're usually so caught up in the practical organisation and planning of details that are associated with running Fit to Drive, such as training or organisational planning, that the discussion of core questions, such as educational messages, are conducted in the context of preparation of teaching materials, or production of public documentation. Since the early developmental work on the program there has rarely been time to approach this in a thorough, systematic way. Often educational resources have been introduced without our having had an initial opportunity to view them together. It tends to be during the course of several viewings that we refine and articulate our thoughts about them. One of the regular issues that crop up is the way the young driver problem is framed, along with the messages embedded in the learning activities and presentations. A slight shift in emphasis, the way we frame a question, seems, to us, to alter the intent and the way a message may be received. Slogans may be seen to give an ambivalent message. For example some concern was expressed about the concluding line of the police presentation: '*Your life; your choice*', which could be read as an individualised message that ignores the dimension of responsibility to and for others.

What's worrying us about this MFB presentation? It all seems so wretched, with the stark characteristics of tragedy: the apparent randomness of events. 'It's just one of those things that's all gone wrong' comments one MFB trainee at the end of the case study analysis. Human flaws seem to render rational choices problematic. Nature (the rainy night) conspires to add to the potential for tragedy (the pathetic fallacy).

'It's more Aeschylus' I say, referring to the ancient Greek tragic dramatist, 'when what we are seeking is Aesop'. Graham gives a laugh of surprise and acknowledgement. 'I always loved Aesop's fables!'

Here's the rub.

'It's just one of those things that's all gone wrong': fear and pity and the Monavale story as tragedy

The reference to Aesop's fables is an expression of the search for a clear causal relationship between intention, action and consequence, uncluttered by complex human exigencies, such as loyalty, obligation, pragmatism. The shared need for clarity and order, a clear moral position. In the world of Aesop's fables (Aesop 2008) the unambiguous moral lesson is summed up in the narrator's concluding sentence. In effect: 'If you act in a way that we know to be dangerous and stupid, you will come to a sticky end.' It is a morally satisfying lesson, largely devoid of complexity, or emotion. One person's bad decision and irresponsible behaviour inevitably leads to grief. In the same vein there is a caution that regularly appears in road safety messages: 'More than 90% of all crashes are caused by human error' (European Commission 2012). The message is clear. Eliminate human error and the number of crashes will be reduced. But the tone is neutral. The issue abstracted from the complexity of human lives it is representing. There is no subject with whom the audience can identify, or empathise.

Fables end in an unequivocal moral lesson. In designing the Fit to Drive workshop strategies there has been a tension between two approaches. On the one hand, the dialogue-based, discovery learning approach, with an open-ended conclusion, trusting young people to work through the moral dilemmas and decisions; and on the other, a clearly didactic orientation, with definite messages and guides to behaviour. Although the program affirms the experience, and values the views and contributions, of the young people, the guiding educational messages are always to the fore. This was reinforced, following a period of grappling with the problem of open-ended, indeterminate conclusions to the group activities, with the introduction of scripted closing lines. This was precipitated by the adaptation of the Fit to Drive program to the training of peer road safety educators in Indonesia (Montero et al. 2009). The need to condense the educational messages for the one-off training situation, where there would be no specific road safety follow-up training or professional development available to the road safety ambassadors, who were expected to implement programs in their own communities, led to the development of clear, succinct concluding statements that could be used as road safety 'slogans' in the workplace and community. Such conclusiveness, in the face of often complex and conflicting impulses and desires, lends a moral dimension that is in many respects a descendant of Aesop's fables.

Tragedy, in contrast, recognises the dynamic interplay of actors and scenario, the complexities of the individual, the historical backdrop, the social forces and network of relationships. Tragedies are replete with random events that ultimately leave bodies sprawled all over the stage, with the survivors lamenting over the loss and waste, and the bystanders struggling to understand, to make sense out of chaos, and puzzling over the futility and folly of human action. And it seems that no matter how we struggle to derive the clear educative, rational and moral lesson from the big stories that frame Fit to Drive, the emotional, the visceral response to catastrophic crashes is akin to that of classic tragedy. Chaos rules.

Chaos makes its entrance in the guise of Fate. There is a strong sense of inevitability that pervades the Monavale story. Reason appears to have no place here. This is an abiding issue taken up by road safety education, which manifests as a site of struggle between Fate and Reason. Reason is exercised in the human capacity to unearth and understand causes of events, and to prevent catastrophe. Countering the view of road crashes as 'random events' (Peden et al. 2004, p. 2), education appeals to an idea of the controllability of events, based on rational action.

This apparent opposition of Reason and Fate is confronted directly in the small group workshop values exercise: 'There's no point worrying about being in a crash. If it's going to happen, it's going to happen.' This statement is put to the students in the values clarification activity, when the young people are asked to stand according to whether they 'agree', 'disagree' or are 'unsure' about this statement. The different responses sit along the spectrum between the two extremes – the acceptance of the 'terrors of reality' (of road crashes) as Fate, or the belief in the power of rationality to understand and control our destiny.

These different responses to driving, road safety and risk can also be understood in terms of the archetypal images at work, which may be located in the Apollonian/Dionysian dichotomy, embodying conflicting human ideals. The Apollonian ideal invokes rational, self-disciplined conduct informed by reason and knowledge, summed up in the wisdom inscribed on Apollo's temple at Delphi: 'The most beautiful is the most just'; 'Observe the limit'; 'Shun hubris'; 'Nothing in excess' (Eco 2004, p. 54). This ideal is the foundation for self-governance and restraint, echoed in the road safety message of another of the stories presented to young people: 'The safest decision is often the most enjoyable.' On the other hand we encounter the Dionysian celebration of the joyous, unrestrained surrender to fate, epitomised in the motto classically ascribed to young people as risk takers: 'Live fast and die young.'[3] Dionysus, as the god of chaos, represents the 'unbridled breach of all rules' (ibid.). Dionysus and Apollo represent, for Eco (2004, p. 55), the co-presence of two antithetical deities – 'the possibility, always present and periodically occurring, of an irruption of chaos into the beauty of harmony'.

Car crashes, and even ordinary scenes of road traffic, can carry apocalyptic associations: chaos symbolised, encapsulated, in the machine. Some car advertising plays on this, representing the car as containing an autonomous, but temporarily captive, power and Dionysian overtones. The *fatalistic* embrace of road trauma as the result of workings of Fate is also evident in individuals' attitude to whether society should view a certain number of road deaths as inevitable, and therefore acceptable.[4] It is significant that the Apollonian ideal of order and injunction to 'observe the limit' was from an early point in Greek culture achieved through the manipulation of numbers: 'The Pythagoreans had a sort of holy dread of the infinite and of that which cannot be reduced to a limit, and so they looked to numbers for the rule capable of limiting reality, of giving it order and comprehensibility' (Eco 2004, p. 61). Numbers, statistics, probability, are the means by which order is imposed on the chaos of road trauma.

The Monavale tragedy seems to defy the capacity of Reason to impose order. The accumulation of adverse circumstances: the designated driver drinking alcohol; the last-minute substitution of the replacement driver; the party parent's failure to notice the remaining boys who need a lift; the attraction between the boys and girls which leads to the boys riding in the boot; the pressure on the young woman to drive against her better judgement; as well as the poor driving conditions, unfamiliar car and other 'risk factors'. All appear to lead, inevitably, to the final scene from which it is difficult to extract a moral message.

Fate, while an over-arching, pervasive presence, is not the sole determinant of what constitutes a tragedy. Aristotle (Dutta 2004, p. 249) set out specific requirements for tragedy that continue to inform our understanding and interpretation of the tradition. Tragedy, according to Aristotle, should imitate events that 'evoke fear and pity. These effects occur above all when things come about contrary to expectation but because of one another.' That is, tragedy involves a reversal in fortune, a radical change in the protagonist's destiny (see also, Boal 2000, p. 36). Tragedy's impact is so profound because it involves situations 'in which sufferings arise within close relationships' (Dutta 2004, p. 252).

Importantly, tragedy acquires its particular power through the audience's identification with the tragic character: 'This is the sort of person who is not outstanding in moral excellence or justice; on the other hand, the change to bad fortune which he undergoes is not due to any moral deficit or depravity, but to an error of some kind' (Dutta 2004, p. 251). That is, a person like ourselves: 'His or her bad fortune should come about not through any inherent immorality but through what Aristotle simply calls an "error" (*harmatia*)' (Dutta 2004, p. 234).[5] The young woman at the centre of the Monavale story is a character who, in the tradition of tragedy, appears to have a good life, personal gifts and fine prospects. Yet she has a *harmatia*, a flaw in her character (Boal 2000, p. 36) that leads to the tragedy unfolding. Her *harmatia* is the inability to resist peer pressure, her failure to act on what she knows to be right.

Tragedy, according to Aristotle, 'should not provide moral satisfaction, because moral satisfaction is incompatible with the effect of pity and fear' (Dutta 2004, p. 234). The *fear and pity* that the audience experiences brings about *catharsis*, variously translated as purification, or purgation of the emotions. Shomit Dutta (2004, p. 232) points out that the Greek 'may be construed as meaning that tragedy brings about, through events involving pity and fear, the purification of such events (rather than the emotions themselves)'. The Monavale story *is* classic tragedy. The combination of events, fatal human errors, the stage left with bodies and shattered lives, a series of 'what ifs', divided sympathies, a confluence of forces that must ultimately lead to the inevitable calamity. We identify with the driver, the tragic figure and her human failings. Even the presence of nature – the dark, rainy night on a forest road – emphasises the drama. So many of the images of crashes seen on news bulletins are of night, the darkness made more intense by the glare of lights punctuating the gloom, rendering the scene even more disturbing and frightening. It's little wonder that, shaking his head, the MFB officer comments: '*It's just one of those things that's all gone wrong.*'

The impact of the Monavale story is established by means of these and other elements familiar from a classic tragedy. It is signalled in the bleak momentum of the story, the recognisable decisive moments where the plot might have veered in a different direction, yet accompanied by the insistent pall of inevitability, the foreknowledge of the tragedy to come. The fatal flaws of the key characters are familiar from classic narratives. Is it too much to cast the owner of the car as Lady Macbeth (urging the driver, against her own judgement, to drive into the night)? Even the comic counterpoint – the boys who 'gallantly' offer to get into the boot in place of the girls, because they are attracted to them – recall comic characters, who provide relief from the tension of the narrative, and at the same time through the contrast in mood and the context of events place the tragedy in high relief. The raucous, carefree scene as the car drives off contributes to the pathos. At the same time, this 'effect' and 'affect' is a consequence of the staging of the tragedy in Fit to Drive. The framing, even manipulation of events to evoke the 'tragic'.

The story presents a clear moral predicament for a number of the characters, but particularly the central character, the young woman who had to step in as driver when the designated driver started drinking alcohol. As such it belongs to a tradition of 'serious literature', which places 'heavy emphasis on creating a complex moral vision, highlighting the complexity and contradiction in the characters' moral situation' (Truby 2007, p. 109). The Monavale story represents just such a complex moral landscape. Each 'character' in the story has a moral decision to make that is framed in the group activity that follows as 'responsibilities' and 'choices'. The story compels young people to think about values and 'right thinking', by asking them to think through the values underpinning the decisions of each character.

Seen as tragedy, the main character in the story commits a fatal error in not asserting what she knows to be right. Not only the dead and injured bodies, but her own decline, her 'fallen' state (she has *fallen from grace*), is at the core of the tragedy. The tragedy is reinforced by the former state-of-grace, the 'might-have-been' potential of the character. The presenter notes that she had been a champion, state-grade netballer, and, as an afterword, that her studies and her sport lapsed, and that she was picked up for drink-driving a year later. These dramatically demonstrated possibilities enhance the audience's sympathy with, and engagement in the fate of the character. Her 'fatal flaw', her *harmatia*, is a lack of moral conviction or strength of character, but it is one the audience may identify with. The extent to which she is, by bowing to peer pressure, *responsible* and therefore not a victim (Truby 2007, p. 127) is often the subject of debate within the workshop groups. Her very lack of self-revelation or insight underscores the pathos of the situation. The loss of the young men is given additional significance by the mention, in the newspaper article, of their 'popular' status – a recurring theme: 'Two mates, Sam Turner,

18 and Billy O'Connor, 17, both boarders in year 12, and *both very popular at school*' (MFB 2006, our emphasis). Their prowess in sport and their success – one had been school captain, with a job lined up overseas – reinforces the point.

So, it *is* classic tragedy – the young woman's life, her being, has been decimated – without the redeeming inspiration the audience might have acquired had we been told of the hero's insight, or self-revelation gained from the experience, something we might see in Shakespeare's *Hamlet*, or Schiller's *Don Carlos*. There is none of the satisfaction of fictional tragedy, where the characters will experience a moment of self-revelation (Truby 2007, p. 40). In the news report, where the court scene serves as a coda for the story, no-one seems to be the wiser. There is none of the dramatic release, or catharsis, of authored story (Boal 2000; Dutta 2004). The audience must step into the drama and become 'actors' or 'chorus' or, more accurately, authors. They get to rewrite the plot, reconsider the choices and make different decisions. If they don't do this, they will be left with an open-ended story. They will be left with all the ambivalence that accompanies tragedy.

The tragedy goes to work: Brandon Glen Secondary College, November 2009

The students head off to their respective rooms with their facilitators. 'Alison's' group are soon settled on the desks and chairs around the room. Alison briefly recaps the circumstances of the crash, then explains that they will divide into four groups to look at the four questions, or issues. She places four signs around the room: 'Choices', 'Responsibility', 'Impacts', 'Peer Pressure', and divides them into four groups, each group to sit by one of the signs. She gives each group some laminated sheets – copies of the case study, and a worksheet to write the group's responses – and tells them they will have ten minutes to discuss their scenario and work out their responses.

As the groups get into the task Alison goes around the room, speaking with each group, clarifying the task and exploring some of the issues. The groups are quite animated and involved, and most of the students contribute their opinion at some point. Some students who appear to be quiet and removed have actually been listening to the others. They come to life to debate a particular point.

After ten minutes or so, Alison calls the group together to listen to the feedback from each in turn. Sitting casually on the table at the front of the room, with the young women still sitting in their groups, leaning against tables, on chairs or the floor, Alison says, with some energy, 'So! we're going to go around the groups, and find out what each group came up with, and discuss the scenario. So we're going to hear from the groups, and if there's anything you would like to say about it, add, change, disagree or whatever, you can say that after they've spoken. OK?'

The divergent orientations to road safety – the possibility of controlling events through the application of Reason, or the random play of dark forces that refuse to order themselves under the rule of Reason – emerge in the individual student responses to the Monavale story. However, the students are not encouraged to linger on the apparently hopeless nature of the scenario, but are instead immediately guided, through the structured activities in the small group session, towards an analytical and solution-focussed working-through of the factors leading to the disastrous crash. The residual impression of the tragic lingers in the themes, notably the inventory of calamitous consequences explored under the theme of 'Impacts'. The idea of the flawed character haunts the 'Choices' theme.

In their responses the students readily pick up on the idea of 'impacts', citing the metaphor of the 'ripple effect'. When the group exploring 'impacts' is invited to report back, the young person speaking for the group explains the impacts for the driver: *'She felt it was her fault, and she lost all of her friends because of it, and now she's a depressed alcoholic. She quit netball because of it. She couldn't finish her VCE. The victim's parents want her in jail. Now she has to live with it forever, and now she's under real stress, and … basically her life has been ruined, because of the pressure of being put into that car.'The boys' families, they lost their sons because of it, and Emma's parents had to support her through the court case because of it.'*

The students refer to the impacts on the broader community: *'And, how the community got affected.'* They draw on their own experience of local community to reinforce this point: *'We all know that when somebody dies from your school everybody at the school gets affected, whether they're close to that person or not … yeah … and those boys were from a small town, everybody would have known them pretty well. It was a pretty prestigious school, so there was big media coverage, and people would have known the parents …'*

The group with the task of discussing 'impacts' finds it hard to ignore the question of responsibility, and the discussion invariably moves from 'impacts' to this: *'And, the other passengers, they were affected, because the designated driver started drinking, so she pretty much bailed on everyone.'* Not only the designated driver, but the owner of the car as well comes under scrutiny: *'The owner, Sarah, she didn't take responsibility, even though it was her car.'* In the context of the Fit to Drive aim of raising awareness of being safe and responsible as a passenger, it is significant that students assert that: *'The passengers should have taken responsibility.'*

As one student relates her group's responses she refers to some of the key people in the story by name: *'If Emma hadn't asked the boys to come along they wouldn't have died.'* This somehow makes it more personal, as if the students identify with the characters more than if it was just 'the girl' or 'the driver'. She names the 'party parents': *'They didn't take proper responsibility to make sure they could get home from the party.'*

Students are ambivalent and even divided over who was responsible, of whether it was a clear-cut matter of an unequivocal case of blame, and therefore, cause. This issue is often hotly debated in the groups. *'The driver made the wrong choice. It was OK to drive but not with so many people in the car.'* The allocation of responsibility and culpability to the driver causes some young people to reflect on the nuances of responsible, and irresponsible, driving: '*Even though she drove irresponsibly because there were too many people in the car, she didn't speed did she? She didn't drink,'* said one student as she grappled with the implications of what constitutes 'responsible' driving.

'Responsibility' is closely tied to 'choice'. Each person in the scenario is seen to have a choice to make, including the young men in the boot: *'The boys made their own decisions to get into the boot. Nobody made them get into the boot.'* While affirming the imperative of responsibility and good decisions the students, when prodded by the facilitator, acknowledge that it is often difficult for an individual to assert themselves in relation to those decisions. The facilitator's question: '*Who's done something stupid because your friends were there?*' is greeted with nods, rueful smiles and grimaces of acknowledgement.

Amid the discussion of responsibility and choice hovers the consciousness of the random nature of events: *'It could have been anyone faced with that – it just happened to be her.'* The facilitator guides this train of thought back to a discussion of peer pressure, leading the young people in reflecting on situations where they had been faced with 'peer pressure'. By recalling similar situations, students can comprehend, 're-experience', the situation of the Monavale driver: 'to comprehend a human experience, whether one's own or that of another, is to bring it into the light of one's own possibilities – and thus to re-enact it' (Todres 2007, p. 10). From this point of immersion in the experience they are encouraged to begin to work through (re)imagined situations, and to think through their own responses and actions if faced with similar dilemmas. In this way once again the story is used as a way of working through everyday situations and decisions, and encouraging the students to plan and rehearse safe choices.

The tragic and the problem of death

Sheila Kitzinger, the renowned feminist who campaigned to change the ways in which the medical profession had come to understand pregnancy, childbirth and antenatal and post-natal care of women and children, died, aged 86, on 11 April 2015. Her obituary in the *Guardian* (Hayman 2015) listed her many achievements, the best-selling books that resonated with professionals and the general public, the posts she held, and the impacts of her work, her life. As Suzie Hayman (2015) wrote, Kitzinger, the 'high priestess of natural childbirth', had done 'more than anyone else to change attitudes to childbirth in the past 50 years'. Kitzinger argued that 'childbirth should not be reduced to a pathological event and she waged a relentless crusade against its medicalisation'. But Kitzinger, suggests Hayman, would also be remembered for the way she lived her life. She was, apparently, 'an intensely likeable woman – warm, intelligent, funny and youthful to the end'; a woman 'unashamed and forceful about being a feminist social revolutionary, her belief centred on the opportunity for women to reclaim their bodies'.

In June 2015 Celia and Jenny Kitzinger, two of Sheila's five daughters, wrote an article for the *Guardian* in which they tried to convey what it meant for their mother to have a 'good death' (Kitzinger and Kitzinger 2015). At the time of her death their mother had 'cancer and many other diseases of old age'. After an initial course of treatment when she was first diagnosed Shelia had 'declined further investigation or intervention'. The Kitzinger sisters noted that their mother had 'spent her life campaigning for autonomy and choice in childbirth and challenging the medicalisation of birth … When it came to dying, she expressed the same values of choice and control, and she planned ahead.' These preparations had included establishing lasting powers of attorney for her health and welfare, and preparing a living will document detailing the sorts of treatment and intervention she would accept or decline. Her aim was to die at home on her own terms: 'Being at home was essential to her idea of a "good death"'. She wanted to be in familiar surroundings, on her own territory, with the support of those who knew her. According to her daughters she particularly did not want to go into hospital, aware as she was of the array of possible interventions that can be mobilised at the end of life, just as when women are giving birth (Kitzinger and Kitzinger 2015).

The sisters acknowledge that the circumstances of their mother's life, her illnesses, and her dying meant that she was able to wrest some control over what had come to be recognised as inevitable. She was dying and her death had a predictable trajectory. But this trajectory, its inevitableness, did not lessen the pain, the hurt, the sorrow that can accompany dying, can accompany death. At the end though these plans, the choices made and shared, the care available, 'allowed Sheila to die, as she had lived, on her own terms. It also allowed us to have positive memories of the last weeks of her life – and that now helps us with our grief' (Kitzinger and Kitzinger 2015). The sisters finish their story with an account of their mother's 'private burial' in a woodland setting, 'without fuss', and accompanied by Sheila Kitzinger's own poetry that captured a sense of peace and silence beyond the pain and suffering.

Not all deaths are tragic. The story of Sheila Kitzinger's 'good death' is not unique, though it is recent, it has some profile, and her daughters tell us something about its unfolding. The story of her dying and death, like countless other such stories, tells us that sometimes death can be a relief, an end to pain, to suffering. Such a death can be called a 'good death'. And a good death can be called a good death because it may come at the end of a good life, a long life. The ways in which a good life and a good death are experienced, are felt, are remembered will be very different to the ways in which a tragic death, even life, is experienced, is felt, is remembered.

Fit to Drive, in telling stories of the road crashes in which young people die, and of the unfolding events that lead to these deaths, and which then echo through families, schools and communities, cannot imagine or understand or use these deaths in any way other than through their 'tragic' character. And it would be very difficult, even crude, uncaring and unfeeling not to agree with the tragic dimensions and consequences of deaths such as these. Young lives.

Cut short. Possibility and potential unrealised. Lives thwarted. Parents grieving. Friends traumatised. Schools and communities in shock. Those who survive, changed forever. A death in these circumstances looks vastly different to the good death that is planned and managed in its inevitability.

What we are thinking out loud here does not, should not, diminish the tragic dimensions of the young lives that are cut short, are lost in these ways. Nor should it be read as arguing that Fit to Drive – in framing a school based health promotion intervention by appealing to emotions, by engaging young people through story, through tragedy, by asking young people to suppose that fate, or crash, or risk can be countered, if not overcome, by reason and rationality – is wrong in understanding young deaths as 'tragic'.

Thinking about death here, the problem of death, should instead be read as trying to open up the many possible dimensions of death. And, by definition, of life, a life. These dimensions are multiple, and complex. And, in thinking of all the possible gradations between a good death/tragic death, good life/tragic life, short life/long life, they are also ambiguous. As our discussion to this point has indicated, many of these dimensions shape the contours of the hinterland from which Fit to Drive emerges. And at different times during the workshop these dimensions are, once again, made present, made manifestly absent, or made absent as Other.

There are, for example, social and cultural dimensions to the diverse ways we imagine and deal with and talk about death. How do we deal differently with different deaths? Is it more 'tragic' if the victim, the young person, is 'popular', 'pretty', 'clever'? Able? Disabled? At various times Fit to Drive brushes up against these dimensions and is troubled, unsettled by the encounter. There are economic dimensions to the problem of dying, of death. What price a life? What costs is a community prepared to bear in relation to safety and the risks of harm and death (vehicle, licensing, road infrastructure)? But also in relation to so many illnesses, diseases, threats to life and the resources that are, or could be, mobilised in relation to these? In the health promotion that Fit to Drive does the economic dimension is largely absent, the space taken up by other ideas, such as 'choices', 'responsibility', 'impacts', 'peer pressure'. There are always, also, political dimensions to death and dying. Do some lives matter more than others? This is a conclusion that is far too easy to draw in looking in too many places throughout human history. What priorities emerge in trying to save some lives, not others? What policy and program and legislative choices can be imagined and made in relation to safeguarding young lives? What is an acceptable number of deaths in road crashes? *(330 – that's not too bad is it?)* On the roads, but also in terms of things such as the sale and consumption of alcohol and other drugs. There are bio-technological dimensions to life, dying and death that take on new characteristics in twenty-first-century, bio-genetic capitalism (Braidotti 2013). What are the limits of life, of death? When does life end, death occur? How much bio-technology should be deployed to prolong life, stave off death? There are ethical dimensions. What is a good life, a good death? Who, or what determines these? There are religious dimensions. What comes next? What is the purpose of life? And, of course, there are the much more mundane, prosaic dimensions of death – though no less important in their everyday nature. The feelings of loss, of grief, of sadness, of relief, of peace, of rest that are experienced at the deeply personal level by partners and lovers, parents, sons and daughters, brothers and sisters, friends and colleagues of the person who has died.

At a fundamental level Fit to Drive is a school based health promotion program that is shaped by death. By the tragic dimensions of young deaths, young lives cut short, and by families and communities traumatised by these deaths. In many respects this is school based health promotion that looks and feels different to health promotion concerns with and about young people's diets, or their sexualities, or their uses of alcohol and drugs. Though the tragic possibilities that can too readily attach themselves to the violence, the abuse or the death that can accompany the uses of alcohol and drugs allows us to imagine affinities across these different concerns. Such affinities may be more immediately apparent when young people's self harm, or suicide, or eating disorders emerge as objects of school based health promotion. Our discussion of the tragic here may make these affinities more apparent, or provoke us to re-imagine the ways in which the tragic dimensions of life, of death, are encountered and engaged with and by young people in school settings. It is in this sense that we want to close here with what the post-humanist philosophy and social theory of Rosi Braidotti (2013) can offer as we encounter the problem of death in school based health promotion.

Braidotti's 'posthuman' philosophy and social theory is positioned in relation to the long tradition in western thought of 'humanism', and its constant companion 'anti-humanism'. In the realm of the posthuman, thinking – such as that done by Donna Haraway (1991), Katherine Hayles (1999) and Braidotti – is opening up spaces in which the idea of human exceptionalism is troubled so that our relations with each other, our relations with the 'nonhuman others (animals, machines, objects, systems, environments)' that share the planet, our relations with the planet, can be re-imagined (Herbrechter 2013). In a review of Braidotti's *The Posthuman*, Stefan Herbrechter (2013, p. 7) argues that Braidotti 'is aware that the posthuman figure is deeply ambiguous and mired in projections of desires or fantasies of domination and disembodiment, as well as anxieties concerning apocalypse and extinction'. In a similar vein to Donna Haraway's (1991) embrace of the figure of the 'cyborg', Herbrechter (2013, p. 7) suggests that Braidotti imagines the posthuman as a 'liberating force' that might engage 'the negativity and thanatopolitical dimension of contemporary biopolitical practices (which include intensive farming, animal mass slaughter, biocapital, data-mining, drone-led wars, hypersurveillance etc.)'. For Herbrechter, Braidotti's 'ultimate desire is to rehumanise, re-member and reinvent the human at the penultimate moment – in extremis – between the familiar humanist "yearning" for human potentiality, and the "frustration" about human reality'. As Braidotti (2013, p. 12) herself argues, 'my interest in the posthuman is directly proportional to the sense of frustration I feel about the human, all too human, resources and limitations that frame our collective and personal levels of intensity and creativity'.

The following, from a section titled 'Posthuman theory of death', is challenging, provocative and unsettling in its own right. But it can also challenge, unsettle and provoke us to think differently about the fundamental problems of life and death and the many and varied ways in which they are made present or absent in school based health promotion. And, importantly, these challenges are not 'morbid' or 'death-fixated'. Rather, they are part of what Braidotti (2013, p. 133) identifies as an 'ethics of productive affirmation'. For Braidotti such an ethics frames a 'different way of handling the issue of how to deal with pain and traumas and to operate in conditions which are extreme, while working to bring out the generative force of *zoe* – life beyond the ego-bound human'. A posthuman theory of death approaches death by, in the first instance, 'introducing some critical distance from the allegedly self-evident value attributed to "Life" in our culture'. As Braidotti (2013, p. 133) argues:

> I live in a world where some people kill in the name of a sacralized 'Right to Life'. I would like to refer to a more lucid tradition of thought that does not start from the assumption of the inherent, self-evident and intrinsic worth of 'life' and stresses instead the traumatic elements of this same life in their often unnoticed familiarity.

Life and death are as one. However much we may wish to deny it neither has meaning without the possibility of the other. To live is to die. To die is to have lived. Well or not. For Braidotti (2013, p. 132) the 'full blast of the awareness of the transitory nature of all that lives is the defining moment of our existence'. This dawning awareness 'structures our becoming-subjects, our capacity and powers of relation and the process of acquiring ethical awareness'. In being mortal 'we all are "have beens": the spectacle of our death is written obliquely into the script of our temporality, not as a barrier, but as a condition of possibility'. In being 'have-beens' that thing that we 'all fear the most, our being dead, the source of anguish, terror and fear, does not lie ahead but is already behind us; it has been'. This sense – denied, suppressed, acknowledged, embraced – suggests that death 'pertains to a past that is forever present', that death 'is not individual but impersonal'. Deeply impersonal in so much as its inevitability has no regard for the ways in which it might be experienced, or felt, or remembered as 'good', as 'tragic'.

This recognition is a starting point for Braidotti. Not a dead-end of dread, or of terror, or of resignation. Rather, it is an opportunity to make present what it might mean to imagine life, if we imagine death in these terms. As she argues, the 'proximity to death is a close and intimate friendship that calls for endurance, in the double sense of temporal duration or continuity and spatial suffering or sustainability' (Braidotti 2013, p. 32). In this sense: 'Making friends with the impersonal necessity of death is an ethical way of installing oneself as a transient, slightly wounded visitor. We build our house on the crack, so to speak.' Making a home, a life, here, under these terms, means that we 'live to recover from the shocking awareness that this game is over even before it started'. Our ever-present 'proximity' to death, to its possibility, its inevitability, 'suspends life, not into transcendence, but rather into the radical immanence of "just a life", here and now, for as long as we can and as much as we can take' (Braidotti 2013, p. 32).

Such a view of life, of death, will be deeply troubling for many who see in life, and, ultimately, in death the possibility of transcendence; who will hope, will wish, that there is more to life, more to death. There will be others not looking for transcendence, but who hang on to the possibility of a purpose to life and death that can be found, can be made real. Again, our purpose here is not to solve the problem of life, of death. What Braidotti offers, for us, are a series of provocations that emerge from taking seriously the challenges and opportunities of wandering in the hinterlands from which Fit to Drive emerges. These wanderings aren't without purpose. Indeed, we could, with more time and space explore what it is that Braidotti (2013, p.132) is suggesting when she sketches the outline of an affirmative posthuman ethics:

> I want to stress instead the productive differential nature of zoe, which means the productive aspect of the life-death continuum. It does not deny the reality of horrors, but rather to re-work it so as to assert the vital powers of healing and compassion. This is the core of the posthuman affirmative ethics …

That is a challenge, however, for another time, another space.

The Monavale story, in the end, is an exceptionally powerful, complex and ambiguous story. Students express a seemingly insatiable demand for stories. '*Give us more stories*' is the regular refrain in the feedback. But the key question here is: what to *do* with those stories? The Monavale story has extra work to do, and it goes to work in an organised, structured, way. The students are brought in with specific tasks. Their job, in part, is to do a kind of 'forensic investigation'. In the small groups the story is dissected, and each element examined in turn. In part the task is to try to re-script the scenario, through the identification of alternative choices and courses of action. The risks contained in the story are the obvious – overcrowding in the car, passengers in the boot, road conditions, time of night – but they are also complex, ambiguous. For example, what is the 'risk' in refusing to drive the car (rejection from friends, leaving friends stranded) compared with the possibility of crashing and the severity of the consequences of a crash in the overcrowded car?

Through the combined effect of the analytic order imposed by the activity and the group's dissection of the scenario and characters, the young people are guided to seek to impose some sense of order, a narrative of causation on the story. They dissect the circumstances leading up to the crash, debate the moral choices, and identify alternative courses of action. Wrapping up the activity, the facilitator comments: '*All this stuff is interconnected – choices here, peer pressure there … responsibility. You can't look at just one element without it relating to another.*'

The Monavale story has the power to ignite the imagination and empathy of the students, to excite debate and contradictory feelings and reactions, and to linger in the thoughts long afterwards. A significant element of the power of this story is its resonances with the archetypical features of tragedy present in the Western literary traditions. But it would seem that the weight of the tragic dimensions of the Monavale story has potential to undermine the positive educational message of the session. Without the work that the students undertake in the next session, which aims to help students develop personal strategies, the abiding effect of these elements added together threatens to be overwhelming. The events unfold as the helpless spectator looks on. The lasting impression: '*It's just one of those things that's all gone wrong.*' In school based health promotion it is intensely problematic to leave the complex, the ambiguous, unresolved. There needs to be 'closure', enclosure, containment. But life and death are not always like that.

Notes

1 Zero Blood Alcohol Concentration (BAC): a requirement for inexperienced drivers in graduated licensing systems.
2 In the morning workshop small groups of young people struggled to keep increasing numbers of tennis balls in the air, tossing them to each other as distractions were introduced.
3 Originally quoted by a character in the 1949 movie *Knock on Any Door*, this phrase entered the language as an expression emblematic of the recklessness and live-in-the-moment nature of youth.
4 One MFB officer at the training session described above, when viewing the statistics, and the decline of the number of road deaths in Victoria over the past forty years to a plateau of around 330 annually, put the question to the police road traffic educator: 'What is an acceptable number of deaths? 330 – that's not too bad – is it?' Since that time, the road toll has declined further to 287 deaths in 2011 (Transport Accident Commission 2012).
5 The 'error' or 'flaw' can be an error resulting from ignorance, an error of judgement, a flaw in character, or a sin (see, https://en.wikipedia.org/wiki/Hamartia).

7 Young people as choosing agents?

The dangerousness of risk[1]

Robert Castel (1991, p. 281) argues that in the latter part of the twentieth century there was a shift in the tactics of 'preventive strategies of social administration' which indicate a fundamental departure from the 'traditions of mental medicine and social work'. Broadly constructed, these strategic innovations in the practices of regulating populations involved a dissolution of 'the notion of a *subject* or concrete individual, and its replacement by a diverse combination of *factors*, the factors of risk'. Where risk and the identification of risk factors emerge as a dominant technique for regulating populations then the practice of 'intervention no longer takes the form of the direct face-to-face relationship between the carer and the cared, the helper and the helped, the professional and the client'. Rather, there is a displacement of the face-to-face relationship by an emerging practice grounded in the 'collation of a range of abstract factors deemed liable to produce risk' with regard to certain behaviours and dispositions of a given population. The emergence and power of these practices is, further, connected to changed processes of 'responsibilisation' and regulation of various forms of expertise (Burchell 1996). Here, imperatives of *efficiency* and *accountability* work to position the 'specialists' (the *psy* counsellors, the social and youth workers, the teachers) as 'mere executants'; interpreters of abstracted knowledge generated at a distance via the practices of other forms of expertise and collated and prioritised as a range of factors.

Castel (1991, p. 283) argues that nineteenth-century psy discourses imagined risks in terms of the 'danger embodied in the mentally ill person capable of violent and unpredictable action'. Dangerousness, in this sense, was a 'rather mysterious and deeply paradoxical notion'. In the first instance dangerousness evoked a 'quality immanent to the subject (he or she is dangerous)'. In the second instance it was a quality that is a 'mere probability, a quantum of uncertainty'. As Castel (ibid.) argues, 'there can only ever be *imputations of dangerousness*, postulating the *hypothesis* of a more or less probable relationship between certain *present* symptoms and a certain act *to come*'. For classical psychiatry this technique was subject to a 'double limitation'. One rested on the imputation which grounded the diagnosis of the *dangerous* individual. The second was grounded in the fact that a diagnosis of future *dangers* rested on a prior intervention. That is, an individual had already to be identified as *dangerous*, to be under surveillance (treatment) in order to be thought of as presenting some future *danger*.

In the context of nineteenth-century sanitary and social reforms, imagining dangerousness in these terms was problematised via rationalities of *prevention* and *intervention*; rationalities which began to examine the '*frequency* of mental illnesses and other abnormalities among the most disadvantaged' populations. These calculations were then related to the 'living conditions of the subproletariat – malnutrition, alcoholism, housing conditions, sexual promiscuity' (Castel 1991, p. 284). These moves, argues Castel (1991, pp. 284–285), marked the emergence of a rationality that sought to construct the problems and the techniques of intervention in terms of '*objective risks*: that is to say, statistical correlations between series of phenomena'. There was a shift here to 'reason in terms of risks rather than dangers'. Castel (ibid.) argues, however, that this problematisation of the practice of preventing social ills was limited by the lack of 'specific techniques' able to render this form of regulation operable. While there were tendencies to think in terms of 'populations at risk', or to conceive prevention in terms of 'generalized moral treatment', these practices of intervention continued to be structured by the necessity to 'enter into contact with and take responsibility for individuals'. Prevention of certain future *risky* or *dangerous* practices still rested on the rehabilitation of previously identified and treated individuals subject to ongoing surveillance and intervention. These limitations to preventative, interventionist practices in the psy sciences, in social and youth work, in the 'care professions' are reduced, argues Castel (1991, p. 287), 'if one breaks this *direct* relation with the assisted subject'. This break is enabled by rendering '*the notion of risk … autonomous from that of danger*'. This shift signals the emergence of a rationality that conceives of a risk as not 'arising from the presence of a particular precise danger embodied in a concrete individual or group'. Rather, the risk, in this sense, is the 'effect of a combination of abstract *factors* which render more or less probable the occurrence of undesirable modes of behaviour'.

Castel (ibid.) illustrates the form that these new practices of prevention can take through an analysis of a French system for the 'automated' management of mothers and infants. This computerised technique was based on the practice of 'systematic examination' of mothers and infants (at a few days, a few months and two years old). These examinations aimed to collect data on 'all possible abnormalities of child and mother, whether physical, psychological or social'. The collected data were computerised and organised by risk factor type. Computer generated correlations alerted a specialist (social/health worker) who was:

> sent to visit the family to confirm or disconfirm the *real* presence of a danger, on the basis of the *probabilistic and abstract* existence of risks.

> One does not *start from* a conflictual system observable in experience, rather one *deduces* it from a general definition of the dangers one wishes to prevent.
>
> (Castel 1991, pp. 287–288)

Nikolas Rose (1996) and Gordon Tait (1995) express some concerns about the dangers which Castel (1991) identifies in this transition 'From Dangerousness to Risk'. Tait (1995), for instance, senses a move to mobilise a *social control* view of government in Castel's (1991) argument that:

> 'Prevention' in effect promotes suspicion to the dignified scientific rank of a calculus of probability. To be suspected, it is no longer necessary to manifest symptoms of dangerousness or abnormality, it is enough to display whatever characteristics the specialists responsible for the definition of preventative policy have constituted as risk factors.
>
> (Cited in Tait 1995, p. 128)

For Tait (1995, p. 128) this view of the potentially 'limitless imposition of the unwanted forces of government' misses the productive capacity of at-risk discourses in which the mobilisation of risk emerges 'as a means of equipping the population with new attributes (or equipping a new, wider population with such attributes)'. Rose (1996, p. 17) too questions the prospect that risk, as technique of regulation leads, unproblematically, to the 'totalization … of surveillance, with the prospect of the prophylactic assignation and guidance of individuals to certain paths in a kind of rationalized dystopia'. Rose argues, instead, that risk (assessment, management and prevention) can (might well) provide a technique for responsibilising the activities of diverse forms of expertise, through, for example, legal and administrative sanctions for *failing* a duty of care: *You should have been aware of the risks.*

However, as we have argued elsewhere, these are *dangerous* times (Kelly 2001, 2013). A dangerousness indicated by the apparently widespread sense of *unease, anxiety* and *uncertainty* in Anglo/European liberal democracies. Here uncertainty attaches to the future outcomes for/of the planet, the nation state, national (mono/multicultural) identity, the economy. And, for young people in particular, to relationships, diet, sexuality, gender relations, the self. When the ('limitless') possibilities for government that risk techniques promise are situated in the context of the transformations structured by processes of reflexive modernization, and of globalisation, the *dangerousness of risk* (the risks of risk), become more evident. Particularly in the regulation of youth as a population constructed in terms of transitions to preferred (ideal) futures, and historically, as emerging from the ungovernable 'wild zones' of modernity's imaginings (Kelly 1999). Here the enhanced capacities for (electronic, computerised, audio/visual) surveillance of populations, developments in biogenetic (social) engineering, the possibilities of/for *cyborg* futures, and the global flows of signs and spaces structure new spaces and relations in which regulation can occur.

It is in this sense that Castel (1991) well captures the dangerous possibilities provoked when, as Rose (1996, p. 20) argues, 'we allow all cultural practices to be "vivisected at the micro-level" and give our experts the duty of defining and managing them in order to eliminate or minimize any possible features that might prove dangerous'. For Castel (1991, p. 289):

> The modern ideologies of prevention are overarched by a grandiose technocratic rationalizing dream of absolute control of the accidental, understood as the irruption of the unpredictable. In the name of this myth of absolute eradication of risk, they construct a mass of new risks which constitute so many new targets for preventive intervention. Not just those dangers that lie hidden away inside the subject, consequences of his or her weakness of will, irrational desires or unpredictable liberty, but also the exogenous dangers, the exterior hazards and temptations from which the subject has not learnt to defend himself or herself, alcohol, tobacco, bad eating habits, road accidents, various kinds of negligence and pollution, meteorological hazards, etc. Thus, a vast hygienist utopia plays on the alternate registers of fear and security, inducing a delirium of rationality, an absolute reign of calculative reason and a no less absolute happiness for a life to which nothing happens. This hyper-rationalism is at the same time a thoroughgoing pragmatism, in that it pretends to eradicate risk as though one were pulling up weeds. Yet throughout the multiple current expressions of this tranquil preventive conscience (so hypertrophied at the moment in France, if one looks at all the massive national preventive campaigns), one finds not a trace of any reflection on the social and human cost of this new witch-hunt.

In this chapter, taking up some of the challenges and opportunities that Castel's thinking provokes, and the broader critiques of the question of agency and of structure, the individualisation of risk and the notion of 'choice biographies' that continue to trouble youth studies, we explore the implications – the complexities and dilemmas, as well as the benefits – of positioning young people as 'choosing agents' in relation to road safety. These challenges also speak, more generally, to a whole range of concerns with young people's health related behaviours and dispositions. We will explore whether, in the context of the social, economic and cultural realities that shape, and necessarily limit choices, this is a constructive way of thinking about individual (young people's) agency in the context of health promotion, but much more broadly in the context of a globalising, neo-liberal understanding of personhood (Kelly 2014, 2013).

The chapter discusses and analyses the second facilitated small group workshop as the Fit to Drive program takes up the idea of young people as having agency to exercise choice, and to act upon that choice. In the first small group discussion session of the Fit to Drive workshop the students tease out the Metropolitan Fire Brigade (MFB) crash study into elements that, separately, can be analysed and debated. They start to consider the possibilities of alternative choices in situations that put them at risk. They explore the ways that choices are made in the roiling current of obligations, allegiances, loyalties and negotiations of the friendship group. In the second small group session the aim is for the students to apply the learning, to prepare themselves for situations when they will need to act, and to speak up, to make themselves safe, and possibly to influence their friends. To exercise what Fit to Drive and so much of youth focused practice, intervention and education imagines as 'agency'.

This section of the workshop consists of two activities. The first ('A closer look at risk') aims to reinforce and apply the learning about the types of situations and behaviours that put young people at risk of harm on the roads. The 'A closer look at risk' activity involves the students in exploring specific risks associated with driving and reinforces the idea that driving is inherently risky, but that certain behaviours increase the risk, that is, the likelihood, of a crash.

The second activity is a problem-solving and role play exercise where students develop strategies to get out of unsafe situations, and practise the behaviours and language they will need to be able to draw upon to manage this. The 'Scenarios' activity is viewed as the key opportunity to bring together the learning gained in the workshop. The young people are asked to respond to scenarios describing risky driving situations, with the scenarios representing familiar situations involving dangerous driving contexts and peer influence. Building upon their understanding of the factors that place them 'at risk' of being involved in a crash, they develop strategies to deal with those situations. The participants are also asked to think of phrases that they could use when demonstrating assertiveness skills, and to practise those phrases within the group.

Talking about and rating the risks

> We all have choices.
>
> (16-year-old female student)

> I learnt about 'choices' and the power of the word I.
>
> (17-year-old male student)

> [I learnt] risks involved in driving and strategies to minimise risk and the importance of letting others know of risks.
>
> (16-year-old female student)

> There are risks in all situations.
>
> (16-year-old male student)

The following account of the first part of the second small group session is taken from a workshop held in Cook College, an all-girls school in a large regional city in Victoria. In the first part of this account the facilitator, Chrissy, works to energise the group to engage them in the next activity after the extended discussion in the MFB case study.

'I want your attention!' calls Chrissy across the din. She divides the participants into three groups, numbering them off, 'one, two, three' and directing each group to a corner of the room. Once groups are divided and are seated on the floor Chrissy announces 'I've got in my hand three sets of risk cards, which I'll give to each group.' She hands each group a set of cards. 'Each of these cards depicts a driving activity. As a group you must line them up in order – so place your cards down from what you believe is the most extreme risk to a high risk of having a crash. Any questions?' There are none, so the small groups set to their task, working together to consider and evaluate their order of cards. Chrissy advises them to 'stick with your instincts'. In each group there are a couple of leaders, taking cards, showing them and consulting with others in the group, and laying them down in a ladder formation. Some groups start to put a couple of the cards next to each other, in a line, within the ladder formation, and there's much discussion as they pick up cards, place them down, and then change their minds again. By this time there are many voices clamouring to be heard in the group.

After about five minutes of working on the task of prioritising their cards, Chrissy gets the groups to come into the middle and line their cards up against each other in the order that they had decided, to compare each group's results. She gets everyone to stand in a circle around the cards to discuss and review the ranking as a whole group. Inviting them to explore the risk in each card, she asks their reasons for their ranking, posing the question 'What is the risk in this card?' or inviting them to 'talk me through your reasoning here'. She leads the group in questions and discussion, first around the question of 'driving without a licence'. 'What is the situation if you are driving without a licence?' she asks. Responses from the students include 'reckless driving', 'inexperienced', 'showing disrespect for the law'. Chrissy picks up on other cards: 'Driving a stolen car. What's the risk in that?' Students: 'It's crazy.' It involves 'reckless driving'. 'It's dangerous.'

Now it's time to complete the final activities. Having organised the students into three small groups to rank a number of driving-related 'risk' cards, Chrissy has brought them back together to discuss their rankings:

Question from student: 'When you talk about dangerous – do you mean dangerous as in you're going to have an accident and die? Or dangerous as in penalties – 'cause, driving a stolen car, you could be a perfectly good driver, you just happen to be driving a stolen car.' Chrissy unpacks this question and challenges the group to think about the likely circumstances where someone might steal a car, the fact that they're already engaging in something illegal, the anxiety and adrenaline levels involved. Someone, she notes, had mentioned 'risky'.

'The term risky – what do you think risky is?' asks Chrissy. 'Causing an accident, getting in an accident' is the reply. 'So,' continues Chrissy, 'is that

how you judged it – the likelihood of killing yourself, or hurting yourself, or hurting other people?' Emphatic nods and agreement from the group: 'Yep.'

A student goes back to the risk of driving a stolen car: 'It would be speeding, extremely risky.' Another girl, 'They wouldn't be used to driving the car.' Another student muses, 'I guess it should be driving dangerously with a stolen car, rather than driving a stolen car.' There's further discussion about this, and another student thinks, 'I guess if you're driving a stolen car, there would be the whole adrenaline factor, you wouldn't be worrying about being safe.'

A girl decides to move the 'Driving a stolen car' card up to the top of the ranked cards.

Another student has been considering the ranked cards. 'I think driving while tired should be way up there.' 'Why?' 'I dunno, I just think it's really dangerous ... just as dangerous as if you've been drinking.'

Chrissy: 'Do you remember the police presentation? When you've been awake 18–20 hours it's equivalent of driving at .05. So, fatigue is one of the biggest killers on the roads.'

Someone moves the cards again: 'I reckon it should be up here.'

The students continue to pick up on the different card scenarios. 'Driving without a licence – is that, like you're on your L's, or driving if you've lost your licence?' 'Driving too close to the car in front of you.' A discussion of braking times follows this.

'Carrying unrestrained passengers.'

'Why are unrestrained passengers such a big deal?' asks Chrissy. 'Because they can fly through the windscreen, around the car,' someone replies.

'And also,' adds Chrissy, 'unrestrained passengers tend to move around in the car a lot'. She mimes this comically 'Yay! Change the radio – yeah! Reach over and grab the lollies out of my bag, yeah, gonna do this, gonna do that – People running around in the car (as much as they can run around in the car) is not a good thing, in such a small space.' Chrissy uses humour a lot, which the girls seem to enjoy and respond to.

A discussion follows about driving and talking with passengers, but soon it's time to wind up the activity – there's still another to do – and Chrissy moves to summarise the discussion and reinforce some of the key points. She refers to an information sheet which provides her with some statistics and analysis. She confirms the risks of each of the cards that have been ranked by the groups as the most extreme. Pointing her toe at the top of the cards, she declares: 'Really extreme risks. BAC 0.15, speeding in a built-up area, driving a stolen car. Why?' She shoots the question to the group. And just as quickly come the answers, which Chrissy validates by repeating: 'Adrenaline, driving like an idiot, trying to get away – well, I'm just assuming, I've never driven a stolen car.' Laughter.

Chrissy concludes the discussion with a bright 'Thanks for your work guys! So, we've learnt that these cards all contain an element of risk. We need to be aware of these risks when we're driving or in someone's car.'

'A closer look at risk' was originally part of an earlier program ('Survival on the Roads'). The activity, then called 'Rating the risk', was designed, in consultation with road safety advice from VicRoads, to generate group discussion about the risks associated with driving, and to specifically incorporate the idea that some driving-related behaviours carried a greater *objective risk* than others. The mildly competitive element introduced by the comparison of small group ranking orders created a high level of engagement with the content. With the introduction of 'Rating the risk' to the Fit to Drive workshop, the activity was adapted to accommodate the need to condense the learning within the time constraints of the school program. One of the changes was to reduce the number of 'risk cards' so that a number of 'low risk' driving situations were discarded (for example, 'a 45-year-old driving at noon' – there is a statistically low risk of crashing when compared with the other scenarios). The remaining cards were mostly categorised as carrying a notable degree of risk. The learning focus in these sessions is on the discussion that occurs when the small groups are brought back together following their attempts to solve the ranking order of the different driving situations according to level of risk. In the original version the facilitators would focus discussion on why one activity is rated as 'most extreme risk' when compared with another activity of 'lower risk', and would offer a solution from an 'official' version, with explanatory notes on why a particular behaviour or scenario was deemed to be a high risk: for example, 'Driving with a BAC level of .15 increases the chances of being involved in a crash by 25 per cent'.

As the revised version was introduced to the workshops, however, the conduct of the activity became problematic for the facilitators. Feedback from facilitators conveyed their confusion about how they should conduct the activity. The idea that one risk can be objectively measured against another, and rated as 'greater' or 'lesser', was called into question. The educational message was considered unclear, and the conclusions the students were drawing from the exercise were misleading and potentially unsafe. For instance, students were taking away the message that they didn't need to exercise care with regard to some of the lower-ranked activities (such as 'an 18-year-old driving at noon') which were designated as low or medium risk.

The discussion surrounding the conduct of this activity reflects the shifting views about the exercise and even uncertainty about its actual purpose. The feedback from some facilitators reflected uncertainties that emerged in project development meetings, facilitator training, and various attempts to distil the learning objectives and capture the key road safety message, to be expressed in the closing line. The first version of the closing line, which was an attempt to move away from a notion of 'ranking', was the feeble, and also misleading, catch-all: 'These cards all contain elements of risk, just like most things in life.'

The focus on awarding a 'correct' ranking, in this activity, was subsequently abandoned. Essentially, the activity in its current form seeks to reinforce the universal message of the program: driving is a potentially dangerous activity that, unless we exercise great care, leads to injury, disruption to life, and often to death. Certain situations and behaviours increase the likelihood of a crash, and of serious harm. Along with the changes the activity was renamed

'A closer look at risk', a more neutral title that reflects the aim, as described in the 2009 training notes: '[for students to] consolidate their opinions, and the facts they have heard throughout the day, using the relative risks of different driving situations'. To reinforce the message the facilitator training notes cautions: 'Remember that all the cards are RISK cards – **you can never remind them enough about this fact**' (Ariens 2010, original emphasis).

At one level the rethink reflects the program team's developing understanding of the pedagogy of road safety promotion, as well as a deeper engagement over time with road safety research and attempts to understand explanatory accounts of young driver crashes (conventionally couched in terms of 'risk'). At another level the activity also reflects an abiding confusion surrounding understandings of 'risk'. The original version attempted to impose a realist, techno-scientific frame on risk, as an 'object' that is amenable to measurement (Lupton 1999a; Ewald 1991). Against this logic the responses of young people were highlighting a more ambiguous, even ambivalent, relationship to 'risk'. The students' questions, challenges and difficulties with 'ranking' highlight the subjective, socially constructed dimensions of defining risk. The activity itself provokes students to define 'risk' for themselves:

'When you talk about dangerous – do you mean dangerous as in you're going to have an accident and die? Or dangerous as in penalties – 'cause, driving a stolen car, you could be a perfectly good driver, you just happen to be driving a stolen car.'

For this young person 'risk' was immediately translated to 'danger'. In one sense, the activity leads them to conclude that 'risk' is about cause and effect (if you do *that, this* will happen). In another sense, it confronts them with the uncertainty/unknowability of events, and the provisional status of any 'risk assessment'. Throughout the workshop 'risk' is presented as a taken-for-granted concept, but in essence the various uses to which it is put carry different, overlapping, meanings. The 'risk' activities depicted in the cards in this segment of the workshop are presented, and ultimately received as, variations of the likelihood of the occurrence of an event, and the severity of the consequences of such an event. Many of these young people, in their initial approach to the task, appear to interpret 'risk' ('most extreme risk' to 'high risk') in the light of the catastrophic scenes represented by the stories they have heard. In these stories 'risk' is viewed, or experienced, as an amorphous manifestation of disaster. 'Risk', in this sense, is an expression of the most severe consequences of an action. Rarely, at this stage of the workshop, is the risk interpreted by the students as positive (as with earlier responses to the values activity, such as 'it's fun to speed'). The activity itself discourages this interpretation. The underlying assumption in the 'Risk' activity is of 'risk' as being associated with negative events: danger, hazard, potential harm.

This idea of danger is combined with a calculation of the 'likelihood' of an event (crash), and the likely harms caused by the event. For instance, not wearing a seat belt may not directly contribute to a crash in the same way driving while fatigued does, but increases the likelihood of severe injuries or fatalities in the event of a crash. It is also suggested, as Chrissy points out when she acts out the behaviour of distracting passengers, that drivers and passengers who neglect, or refuse, to wear seatbelts are more likely to be negligent drivers, and distracting, or a bad influence, as a passenger. The presence of multiple 'risk factors' compounds the risk, as reinforced by the closing line that was eventually settled upon: 'the more exposed you are to risks on the roads, the greater the likelihood of a crash' (Ariens 2010).

The extended discussion and ongoing refinement of the 'Closer look at risk' activity demonstrates the confusion related to 'risk' and its various meanings. Despite the attempts to make tangible and quantify abstract questions of danger and possibility under the name of 'risk', the word itself continues to wriggle out of the grasp of the various players, characters and participants in the development and conduct of the workshops. The activity can succeed in reinforcing the 'riskiness' of, and need to avoid, certain driving behaviours and situations. However, in an unintended outcome, it can also lead many young people to the conclusion that 'there are risks in all situations' (16-year-old male student, Marymede Secondary College). This is an interpretation that can reinforce a resigned submission to 'fate', the opposite of the intended outcome of the workshop.

The understandings of risk revealed in the discussion session, and expressed in the student evaluation comments at the end of the program, reflect the diverse perspectives and understandings of 'risk' present in contemporary understandings of the word. Students who locate their thoughts about the different 'risk scenarios' in the specific, and contextualised, imagining of their own extended experience often express an ambiguous understanding of the variables present in the scenarios. Their comments draw attention to questions of human agency and capacity to make judgements in the context of complex choices and competing demands. They allude to the possible ethical and moral dimensions residing in the situations represented in the bald statements of the 'rating the risk' cards. Though guided in the 'Risk' activity away from a ranking of the different risks, young people in the workshop reveal through their questions and comments an understanding and acceptance of the notion of hierarchies of 'risk', framed as assessing and weighing – usually undesirable – options: '*What if someone like your mum was dying and you needed to get her to hospital and you didn't have a licence, could you get into trouble with the police for driving her?*' (Student question reported back in Locarno College debrief notes, August 2010). The assessment of an 'objective risk', such as speeding, is mediated through the prism of familiarity and habituation: '*My dad's a good driver, though he sometimes speeds.*' Often this is framed as 'trust': '*I trust my brother, even if he's had a few drinks.*'

Ultimately, 'risk' is interpreted, and accepted, by many of the young people in the workshops as being about choice: as a weighing of actions, and an assessment of likely or potential consequences. The contention that young people are 'at risk' due to inherent factors is occasionally cited by the young people, but is mainly associated with inexperience, rather than putative 'biological' factors. The most pervasive attitude of young people, expressed in feedback and in the course of the workshops, is their acceptance of driving as being dangerous, of crashes being caused by individual behaviours, and a subsequent acceptance of individual responsibility.

Acceptance of the idea of 'risk' as an expression – and enactment – of 'choice' is reflected in the students' comments in group discussions, and in the feedback responses at the conclusion of the program. This acceptance, not unproblematically, aligns with the educational message of Fit to Drive: the imperative to recognise 'risk' and make 'safe' choices. In the comment of one young man we glimpse a developed sense of risk hierarchies, in the balance of personal responsibility ('choice'), and awareness of the imperative to choose – or, more resignedly, settle on – a compromise from a limited selection of circumscribed options: '*Assess your options, decide which route has the least consequences*' (17-year-old male, Penfort School).

'Stop the car! I'm going to be sick!'

The enactment of safe 'choices', which takes place in the complex, ambiguous 'reality' of the social world, requires a set of personal skills, such as decision making, problem solving and assertive communication. The remaining part of the second small group session is a scenario analysis and role-play activity that aims to provide students with the opportunity to explore and practise these skills. The description below is from a workshop at 'Madderlake Secondary College' in October 2009.

Chrissy goes swiftly to the front of the room and bends to reach into her kit, from which she retrieves two laminated sheets. 'One more activity,' she says cheerfully, working to inject some energy into the group. She instructs the students to form two groups and tells them: 'In your groups you have been given a dilemma scenario. These are situations you may or may not be in sometime. What I want you to do, is one person in your group is to read out the scenario, and you as a group are to come up with strategies for how you would deal with this dilemma. Make it as realistic as possible to you and your peers, and your situation. Once you have come up with the strategies, write a phrase of what you would actually say, how you would say it. So, for instance your strategy might be to fake a "sickie", but what would your phrase be for actually saying it? Get it?'

Some of the students make a move, and Chrissy encourages some of the students who are still seated to 'make a bit of a circle'. Some of the boys are organising themselves to move tables. They finally organise themselves into two groups, and settle down to work, the students with the 'scenario' card in each group looking at the scenario, some peering over their shoulders. Others have taken the opportunity to have a chat. Chrissy checks with the group: 'Does that make sense? You guys will have to make a bit of a circle' (arranging the near group). In one group it is one of the boys who is reading out the scenario, casually lolling on the table top; in the other a girl stands in the middle of the group, capturing everyone's attention and reading it out loudly.

The second group seems to be started on their scenario pretty quickly. Group one is slower off the mark. 'It's big groups, so it should be easy,' encourages Chrissy. She works with this group for a while, talking through the scenario again, prompting responses, asking questions. She checks that they know about writing their phrase in the column on the sheet and explains that they will need someone to feed back their answers to the large group.

Group one is discussing the scenario, although some group members are distracted, and the energy is lower than before. Group one seems to have finished and some are looking a bit bored. 'We've finished,' volunteers one of the girls with her hand up. The scribe hands the paper to one of the boys who has requested to look at it. Now the room's quite noisy as this group chats and exchanges pleasantries. It's interesting that some of them are rehearsing with each other the phrases they've come up with.

Group two is contributing to the noise as well, but they're working on the task still, and there appears to be some debate. Chrissy goes over to the group and listens for a bit. She has to work quite hard to keep the groups on track, and focussing on the task. She probes – 'Have you been in a situation like this?' A mix of 'No' and 'Yeah – sort of' in response.

'What are some of your strategies?' asks Chrissy.

The groups work on this for a few minutes more and then Chrissy calls them back together in the large group. She gets the first group to go first, and asks who's going to feed back for the group. One of the boys is holding the sheet already and starts to read out the scenario: 'After having a bad argument with a friend they are driving you home. You notice that they are driving much faster than usual, are too close to the car in front, and are taking the corners way too fast. Your friend is staring out of the windscreen ignoring you. What do you do? What do you say?'

Chrissy checks that the other group has heard, and then invites the boy to continue. 'OK, we've got a couple of strategies – five.' (holding up his fingers) 'One, tell the driver that they look tired, and if it's OK you'll take over driving. So, "You look tired, I'll drive."' 'Yep,' encourages Chrissy.

'Strategy two is just pull a sickie and say, "I think I'm gonna throw up," or something.' 'Yeah, good one' from Chrissy, at the same time as one of the boys in the other group, who immediately approves of this suggestion – 'Good one!'

Chrissy, in the meantime, is writing the phrases the group comes up with on the whiteboard. The boy continues with the strategies, which include working out the argument with your friend, and 'Say you're not comfortable being in the car and you want to get out.' 'Being honest,' notes Chrissy. 'Do you think it would make a difference who you were with?' They discuss this for a bit and move on to the last one: 'Stop to get food or something.' Chrissy affirms this as a good idea, and asks for phrases they would use.

During the feedback the other group members are fairly quiet, though quite alert. They're letting the boy do all the talking on behalf of the group. There is, however, a fair amount of comment and interest from students in the other group.

Chrissy gives the other group a chance to comment, but they have nothing more to add. They affirm the other group's ideas, expanding a little on these. There's some banter and joking between the boys, and Chrissy draws the points together: 'So, being assertive, that's what you're saying, yeah? You're basically preferring to be assertive, say what you think, and feel.' They agree with this, and Chrissy follows up with a brief story about her friend who was in that situation, tried the different excuses, but finally was simply assertive and asked to be let out of the car. 'And that worked,' declares Chrissy. 'You work with whatever works. It does actually happen.'

She thanks the group – 'That's a good list, thanks guys. It's time for another': 'During a particularly boring evening you are hanging out with some friends, having a few drinks, when two of the guys suggest driving to the beach in one of their cars. "Matt" is happy enough to drive everyone – he's only had four or five stubbies[2] *– and everyone else is keen to go along. But you feel uneasy about the plan, and don't really want to go along. At the same time you don't want to seem like a bore. What do you do? What do you say?'*

'So,' begins the student, 'the strategies we came up with are, convince them not to go – just be honest.' Chrissy: 'Yep: so what are you going to say?' 'I don't want to go.' This is greeted with laughter from the group. Chrissy, drily: 'Pretty straightforward.'

The student continues reading from his list: 'Distract them from the idea, using an excuse of some form.' Chrissy: 'Yep.' 'And our phrase was "I don't have any bathers".' There are amusing asides here. Chrissy: 'This is one of the circumstances where it's OK to tell a little white lie – "work tomorrow", etc. etc. Whatever you felt comfortable with.'

The student is getting into the swing of the discussion: 'Before you started drinking, maybe have a designated driver in case you were going to go somewhere … the phrase would be: "Who's alright to drive?"' Chrissy: 'I'm glad you guys thought of that one, because that's preventing that situation from even occurring. You wouldn't even need to get to that point and worry about it. Haven't really thought about that before.' She nods and affirms this as a good idea. She explores some of the conditions where that would work, the issue of negotiating who would decide, etc.

The student continues: 'Convince them to stay where they are.' Chrissy: 'Yep.' Other ideas follow: 'We need to get more people to come.' He dobs in the only girl in the group, who's sitting next to him. 'Maggie wrote: "Single beds for everyone".' There's laughter and a joking interchange between the boy and Maggie, but she looks a bit embarrassed. Chrissy defuses the situation, commenting, 'Whatever works.' She has continued to write up the responses on the board.

There are a few more strategies: 'Convince them to get other forms of transport – taxi.' Chrissy, as the student winds up her feedback, asks: 'That all of them? You guys?' (to other group) 'Any more suggestions?'

Various students feed back some more ideas. One of the girls from the first group, who's been silent the whole time, but watching with interest, contributes:

'Get your parents to drive you.' Chrissy picks up this point and affirms it as a good idea.

'Call someone,' suggests one student. Chrissy: 'Or call someone. Yep, what's another one?' Student: 'Walk.' This leads to a discussion about the need to exercise caution when walking at night, particularly after drinking.

To finish up Chrissy now gets two students to role play one scenario as an angry, reckless driver and their alarmed passenger, and to practise assertive statements. She gets a boy and a girl who are sitting next to each other to move their chairs to the front and puts them 'in role' as the driver (the boy) and passenger (the girl).

Chrissy sets up the roles for the characters: 'She says something that annoys you; you're pretty angry.' The boy looks angry, screwing up his face comically in a grimace, and there's laughter from the group. 'You're starting to feel unsafe, because he's driving pretty crap' (laughter). 'What sort of things are you going to do to make him stop? Let's see what works. You're really angry, stop smiling!' (mock sternly to the boy, who's got a big grin on his face). They laugh again, but start to act out driving recklessly, the passenger being nervous. She tries out some lines: 'I want to go to the toilet!' There's no change. 'Not working!' says Chrissy.

'I'm hungry!' No reaction. The other students are laughing and being a cheer squad for the 'driver'. 'Are you guys helping or egging him on?' asks Chrissy. One of the boys encourages the passenger. 'Use your drama skills!' 'I just want to get out of the car!' Chrissy: 'Do you think any of these would work?' The passenger, miming desperation, announces 'I just pissed all over the floor!' Amongst the laughter at the gross image Chrissy suggests that 'The puke one has worked the best, because no-one wants puke all over their car.'

The students are enjoying this now; even those who were quiet and appeared a bit lethargic are now animated, smiling, and wanting to add to the discussion. Some of the students are saying it wouldn't work, some are enthusiastically supporting the strategies.

Chrissy concedes: 'Some of these wouldn't work for you in these circumstances, but if you are ever in these circumstances, at least you have some ideas, and you can think of your own, that you think would work for you. So, if that one didn't work, just try another one, do you know what I mean. Just do whatever it takes to get out of that situation. Anything you want to add?'

Chrissy thanks the group for their participation, acknowledging that it's been a long session, and that they're going to head back to the auditorium for the wrap-up.

To locate and think about this activity, and its objectives in the overall context of the program, it is useful to recall the logic of the Fit to Drive workshop structure. First, capture the students' attention and engage them with the problem. This is achieved through personal and emotional connection (story): through facts, and analysis of the problem: build the knowledge, create the motivation to make (behavioural) change: and practise the skills needed that will help to bring about that change. In this case, how to identify a situation that places them at risk (in danger), developing solutions to the problem, and acting on that solution. The approach is based on an affirmation, central to much contemporary youth work practice and health promotion, that young people are 'the experts of their own world' (Young 2006, p. 91). In this frame young people, with support, are imagined as being best positioned to identify realistic solutions to everyday challenges. This view must always remain problematic. We will come back to some of the concerns with this view towards the end of the chapter. For now it is enough to observe that it is only in the context of a highly orchestrated, heavily structured workshop/program, facilitated by a significant number of adult 'experts' and near peer facilitators that young people's 'expert knowledge' of their own world, their 'agency' can emerge.

Importantly, it is to have an opportunity to practise speaking the words that they would/will use in similar situations. Much of the point of the scenarios is to rehearse, ahead of time, the answers, responses, the language, that they will need to be able to readily draw upon, when they need to extricate themselves from a dangerous situation. What is it about the actual experiential rehearsal of the words? How is an apparently superficial, usually comic, experience (the 'car' role play) able to imprint itself so powerfully on the memories and join the repertoire of young people's self-conduct? Workshop feedback often specifically mentions this segment as 'standing out' in their minds. As one 16-year-old female student at Dartmouth Secondary College recalled: '*How to negotiate with the driver who is speeding and wouldn't stop*'. A 16-year-old male (Sunnyside Secondary College) responded: '*I learnt what I could say to others while in a car with drunk friends*'. Another young female student remembered: '*[I learnt] to make excuses if you don't want to go driving with someone that's drunk*' (Rosehill Secondary College).

The workshop that we have just described was conducted just prior to the introduction of the 'Rational/Emotional' framework into subsequent workshops. This framework was a technique introduced for the facilitators to use with the young people, as a means of providing a concrete memory aid and trigger to enable young people to think their way out of dangerous situations. The intention was for students to use the information to 'bring down the emotions' in the driver (in the 'Angry driver' scenario; the 'Beach' scenario presents different dilemmas and options for choices). The 'FBC' formula – 'Feelings, Behaviours, Consequences' – provides a way of thinking through the connections between high emotion and automatic (often careless and dangerous) behaviours in response. The appeal to the 'rational' finds resonance with some young people: '*Don't give in to peer pressure – think rationally*' wrote a 16-year-old female student. Students are being taught, through the scenario, to manage the behaviour of others (that is to slow down, or stop, or drive less erratically) with whatever means available. Ideally this should be the model of assertive communication: 'When you do __, I feel __, and __ [name the consequence]'. The workshop provides the opportunity for students to test out the 'feel' of speaking this by creating and testing out responses they could use.

While many young people are adamant that they would be able to use assertive responses in such situations, some young people question whether the phrases would work. They feel that, in their experience, this approach wouldn't have the desired effect. In the role play students will often need to employ the whole repertoire of invented phrases to achieve a shift in the 'driver's' demeanour and behaviour, demonstrating strategies more akin to bargaining, threatening, wheedling and pleading rather than reasoning and asserting. If it feels uncomfortable for observers – and sometimes facilitators – to witness students role-playing the passenger in this decidedly less than ideal model of assertive behaviours, it emerges from the lived reality the young people bring to the situation. A significant challenge here is to recognise (validate) the students' reality, and to affirm the creative solutions they have devised, while further developing those solutions, and sometimes reframing both the strategies and the language.

An example of the work required to achieve this is described in the debrief notes from Loxley Secondary College (June 2010), in which the logistics coordinator suggests ways for working with student resistance to the generation of phrases:

> **Students who say they wouldn't use Scenario phrases:** It's really important that students gain a couple of strategies and phrases that they would use in real-life scenarios. If you have gone through the activity and it comes out towards the end that one or a few students don't think they would use any of the phrases thought of so far, keep prompting to find out what they would say. Directly ask them, 'If you don't think these phrases would work for you, what would?', then write up any further positive phrases. Not everyone may feel comfortable using every phrase, and that is ok. It's about generating as many ideas as possible to provide options. Whilst in the moment it can feel disheartening if they initially say they wouldn't use the phrases, it's actually really positive that they express their thoughts honestly, as it shows they are thinking about themselves in the situations. It then gives you a better chance to help them and keep 'workshopping' it – much preferred than them leaving the room keeping thoughts to themselves and not gaining as much from the program. It is sometimes hard to judge what students gain from the program – even the most 'macho' often gain much more than they let on.

Again, in the structured and institutionalised spaces where this health promotion intervention unfolds, and emerges from, the tensions shaping a sense of young people's 'agency', the demands to manage, to regulate this agency in ways that support the intended outcomes as imagined by the adult/peer experts are made clear by a logistics coordinator at Woodbridge Secondary College (August 2010):

> **Scenarios** It is great to see everyone implementing the new way of doing scenarios and many are finding it beneficial to introduce FBC at the

> beginning of the activity. Just a reminder that FBC is mentioned in the introduction, but is unpacked once you have written the student's phrases on the board. Just be careful to not push FBC so much that students feel that a phrase without FBC in it isn't good. I saw many times today positive strategies and phrases being ignored because they didn't include FBC. If a student suggests a phrase like 'Let's pick up some chicks' for scenario 2, don't ignore it, ask the student why they feel that would work because it may just be a way for them to break the ice and get the driver to laugh which is a valid strategy and therefore phrase. This is just one of many that were not explored but need to be.

The point made here is that the requirement to bend the students' personal responses and strategies to fit the 'Feelings, Behaviours, Consequences' formula, (which may or may not find a connection within their thinking) carries the potential for overlooking the creative and pragmatic 'solutions' and phrases generated in the group.

While 'peer pressure' is commonly recognised as a factor that contributes to young people's exposure to potential harm – and the need to assess 'risk' within the social reality of peer relationships and allegiances is a genuine concern – an even more problematic dilemma for some young people is how to handle situations where a parent is driving dangerously. Facilitators have frequently encountered students who express greatest concern and sense of disempowerment in the face of parental driving behaviours and attitudes. Accounts of parents driving dangerously, speeding or driving under the influence of alcohol and other drugs include situations when young people have reason to be fearful of expressing their concern or fear, as debrief notes from Dartmouth Secondary College (November 2010) indicate:

> In debrief we had an interesting discussion about phrases in **scenarios with parents**. A student implied that they sometimes find themselves in uncomfortable situations in cars with a parent, and was concerned that some phrases could make them angrier. We brainstormed some ideas and discussed that as well as using the 'FBC' formula, parents might respond well to facts and statistics. Also, by relaying the message from an authority figure (for example stating that 'a police presenter told you …') it may hold more weight from the view of the parent, as the source is credible. Highlighting the issue that's making them uncomfortable by asking for the parent's opinion about it may encourage them to think about their behaviours as well.

Karl Weick (1995), in his work on sense making in organisations, talks about the role of language, and specifically the importance of shared vocabularies, in sense making. Introducing the students to a shared vocabulary of road safety, of which 'risk' forms such a central part, is an integral aspect of the Fit to Drive project of collective sense making in relation to driving. Extending this idea further, Weick (1995, p. 109) observes that 'language transformation can be a pathway to behavioural transformation'. From this perspective, the creation of, or shift to, a common language (vocabularies) can be part of the foundation building for behavioural change. For Gadamer (2006, p. 389) the creation of a common language is fundamental to the 'very act of understanding and reaching agreement'. Language is the form in which understanding is achieved. In this process 'words matter', as Weick (1995, p. 106) observes. The process of creating a common language encompasses – crucially – the language of 'risk'.

Words, language, also contain the capacity for obfuscation, perpetuation of confusion, talking at cross purposes, and false, even conflicting, assumptions and conclusions. Inherent in the dialogue based practice of the facilitated workshops is the possibility that confusion, doubt, dissonance and inconclusiveness will prevail, which may lead to 'negative' ideas, dangerous messages and resistance to the educational message. 'Dialogue is always dangerous', notes Augusto Boal (2000, p. xvii):

> because it creates discontinuity between one thought and another, between two opinions, or two possibilities – and between them infinity installs itself; so that all opinions are possible, all thoughts permitted. However, this fluidity and openness to the possibilities are crucial for the development of understanding that is a result of true dialogue: 'When Two have ceased to exist and only the Sole Absolute Thought remains, creation becomes impossible. Dialogue is democracy.

In Fit to Drive the pedagogical intent is constantly in view: to shepherd the young people towards a defined understanding of risk in relation to road safety. 'Risk', laden with ambivalence, complexity and confusion, needs to be 'bedded down', the meaning (approximately) settled, in order to achieve the pedagogical objective. In this circumscribed space the young people will be able, are enabled, to explore, debate and create 'solutions' to the problems presented to them in the language of risk. The limitations that may be encountered in this may be (are often) framed as being related to young people's restricted scope for agency, their limited freedom and capacity, within this context, to define the 'problem' and to speak to their own lived experience (more on this later). A conversation with a logistics coordinator (Jodie, September 2011) in which she was asked about whether the imperative of the 'closing line' in the 'values activity' limits to an extent the fluidity, open dialogue and discovery effect of the activity, illustrates this dilemma. She noted that, from the facilitator's perspective, there is always scope for students to explore their views, experience and questions, and to come back at the conclusion of the activity to the key question of values, and the way our values underpin out motivations and behaviours. While the discussion can be, within the time limits of the workshop, relatively free-ranging and open, the crucial point is to keep in mind the goal and intention of the activity. The concluding statement of the 'Values' activity steers a careful path between the gaping precipice of open-ended personal opinion and the immovable cliff face of didactic sloganeering: '*We all have many opinions about road safety. However, there are some road safety facts that may influence our opinion. Let's go hear those facts.*' The 'we' and 'our' here signals an intent to be inclusive, to conspicuously avoid standing 'above' or separate from the group. However, it may be argued that the immediate juxtaposition of 'opinion' and 'fact' reminds the group of the authority of the expert knowledge. What is at issue, however, is the overriding concern to challenge – in a safe manner, what are seen to be unsafe messages (opinions).

The interlinked ideas of individual responsibility for the management of risk and the exercise of personal choice underpin the educational message of Fit to Drive and in turn pervade the students' responses. Students' evaluation comments consistently reflect a ready acceptance of the idea of individual responsibility, both in general statements: '*Never let people pressure you into anything,*' writes a 17-year-old female student from Lynton Catholic College; and articulation of specific personal strategies: '*Plan a designated driver,*' suggests a 17-year-old male from Penfort College. '*Speak up if feeling unsafe,*' recommends a 16-year-old female from Meadowbrooke Secondary College. Other students carry the ideas further to think about personal strategies to take into their family and social world: '*Leaving early for a commitment is important so that you don't have to rush like a madman … I wish my whole family could watch this and be safe*' wrote a 15-year-old female student from Lynton Catholic College. Other students highlighted the experience of practising the words to use when negotiating with friends, family and peers: '*[I learnt] what you would say to try and stop your friends driving when influenced by alcohol,*' reported a 16-year-old female student at Loxley Secondary College. Some students are unequivocal in their apportioning of responsibility: '*If you're not comfortable get another form of transport*' insists a 16-year-old female student from Sapphire Gully Secondary College. The persistent expression of individualised responses to road risk in the workshops and student feedback is not surprising, given the educational aims and messages of the program. For those alert to the complexities of the notion of 'choice', however, it is an interesting manifestation of the students' internalisation of individualised risk imperatives.

Beyond agency in health promotion with young people?

Early in Richard Flanagan's (2013, p. 3) Booker prize winning novel, *The Narrow Road to the Deep North*, the main character Dorrigo Evans recalls his mother's sense of what it is to live, to experience life, to accrue memories, to imagine the world and her place in it. For Dorrigo's mother there is a greater timescale and cycle to life than we, as short lived humans, usually appreciate. And that, in many respects, the things that unfold in that cycle *just are*. Are beyond the scope of human intervention. Beyond human agency.

We go looking in young people for that thing we call agency when we imagine that the world doesn't have to just be as we encounter it, as it shapes us, as it sets limits and possibilities. We look to young people to be acting in and on the world in ways that we imagine signify or suggest that thing that we call agency, that thing which suggests a special, purposeful way of being, thinking, doing, acting in and on a world that doesn't have to be just as we find it. It is the special character of this purposeful way of being and thinking and doing that is most problematic for youth studies researchers who are on the lookout for such things. Because that thing that they/we call agency is so special it is not to be found in the everyday, the mundane, the myriad acts of daily life/survival. To be special, to be agency, it has to be something else. And if the being and thinking and doing is everyday, mundane, not special, it can't be that thing that they/we are looking for. It can't be agency. But it is in the everyday, mundane acts that the experience and meaning and limits and possibilities of a life emerge, are encountered, are responded to, are made.

If a tree falls in the forest and nobody sees or hears it, does it still fall? If a young person thinks and acts and does, and a youth studies academic, youth worker, health promotion facilitator doesn't witness it or record it or write about it, does the young person still think, act, do?

The question here then is not one of young people's agency, but one of the making, the assembling of thinking, acting and doing into something we can 'recognise' as agency. As Ian Hunter (1993, p. 129) has argued:

> If by agency we mean human capacities for thought and action then, given the irreducible positivity, variety and dispersion of the technologies of existence and conducts of life in which such capacities are formed, it is implausible to assume that agency has a general form; and it is even more implausible to identify this general form with that special Western conduct that we call the formation of the subject.

So, what might be the limits and possibilities of understanding things such as a choice and agency in doing health promotion with young people? What weight do we attach to the words that are uttered by young people in these contexts, in the Fit to Drive workshop and elsewhere, where young people's 'authentic voice' and 'agency' and 'expertise in their own life' are understood as being central to developing their capacities to make better choices? There are a variety of intellectual resources, a variety of 'thinking technologies' (Haraway 2008), that we could draw on to explore the limits and possibilities that ideas about agency and choice and structure play in much youth studies, much youth work, much youth health promotion. For example, in relation to the ways in which a particular 'right way' of thinking, doing and acting, a preferred form of 'agency', is embedded in Fit to Drive, is embedded in all health promotion programs in schools, we could provide a poststructuralist reading that would highlight, and explore, and critique the power relations, the roles of expertise, the institutional settings that are in play in these contexts. Such a reading would not think in terms of these as, somehow, 'restricting' agency, as structures that limit agency. Rather, what would be of interest are the limits and possibilities of thought, action, imagination, in this always constrained field of possibility. The health promotion space is, in this sense, 'productive' of certain ways of thinking, doing, acting, being (Kelly 2014, 2013).

Debates about structure and agency have formed the core of much work done in youth studies, youth work and health promotion over a long time. In drawing this chapter to a close we want to review aspects of these, ongoing, debates to open up the ground on which some of these concerns might be more fruitfully engaged.[3] A contemporary debate has unfolded in the pages of the *Journal of Youth Studies* (2009–14) between Dan Woodman, Steven Threadgold and Steven Roberts (and others) about the relative merits of the work of Ulrich Beck and/or Pierre Bourdieu for the doing of youth studies. We want to use features of this debate to take up Dan Woodman's suggestion in his contribution to the debate that in quite fundamental ways questions of *agency* and *structure* remain central to significant *uncertainties* (Latour 2007) in the doing of youth studies. Early in Dan Woodman's (2009, p. 243) original *Journal of Youth Studies* article he argued that he was interested in the 'emergence and use of the concept of choice biographies in the sociology of youth over the past decade, a concept that has been called, in critique, a "current pervasive theoretical orthodoxy"'. Woodman (2009, p. 246) then provided a review of the ways in which both the concept of choice biography and, more broadly, the work of Beck has been used and critiqued in youth studies in the last 10–15 years. He spent some time discussing Karen Evans' (e.g. 2007) work on *bounded agency* as a response to a particular reading of Beck's individualisation thesis. For Woodman (2009, p. 246), Evans' approach is representative of a tendency 'to use Beck as a caricature to claim a middle ground between structure and agency'. In these debates about choice, structure and middle grounds, the problem of structure and agency, and the ability of these ideas to make sense of what young people do, and why, remains central (Woodman 2009, p. 247). Woodman (ibid.) argued that while the 'relative balance has swung back and forth, the vast majority of authors within the sociology of youth have proposed some kind of middle ground between agency and structure'. For Woodman (ibid.), occupying some sort of 'middle position between structure and agency also makes sense in light of the way the history of youth sociology tends to be told'. In these accounts of what youth studies has done or should do, a 'structuralist strand of school-to-work transitions research that has been historically critiqued for overemphasizing structure is contrasted to a cultural strand of youth research that is seen to have overemphasized agency' (ibid.).

In early 2010 the *Journal of Youth Studies* published an article by Steven Roberts that responded to Woodman's article. Roberts (2010, p. 137) claimed that his contribution offered a

> response, and some balance, to Woodman's (2009) recent polemic defending the work of Ulrich Beck, and his assertion that those involved in researching the sociology of youth have tended to read Beck incorrectly in a way that promotes young people's lives as being 'choice biographies'.

A key element of Roberts' (2010, p. 145) response was to also provide an account of the concept of bounded agency to map out the so-called middle ground in the structure–agency debate. He argued that, in developing this concept, Karen Evans had demonstrated the 'importance of sociologically analysing the conditions under which actors come to act, insisting that "people act systematically, rather than just idiosyncratically"'. Drawing on the work of Evans and others, Roberts (ibid.) suggested that agency should be understood as a 'socially situated process shaped by the experiences of the past, the chances in the current moment, and the perceptions of possible futures'. Referencing Evans, Roberts (ibid.) indicated that these processes, experiences and perceptions 'manifest "a number of boundaries or barriers that circumscribe and sometimes prevent the expression of agency"'.

According to Roberts (ibid.), 'acknowledging the role that structures play in this middle ground is not the waste of time that Woodman might have us believe'. In this view, structures continue to shape the 'lived experience of young people, and continuing to reveal structural inequality should be part of the repertoire of youth studies because if such inequity continues to exist, then the job is not done'.

Later in 2010 the *Journal of Youth Studies* published a response by Woodman (2009) to Roberts' critique in which he attempted to correct what he identified as a selective reading of Beck and restate his intent to raise questions about the structure–agency debate. The next instalment in the debate came from an article published in the *Journal* in 2011 by Steven Threadgold. Threadgold's contribution was to pitch his tent in the middle ground of the structure–agency debate: a middle ground that for Threadgold (2011, p. 384) is made thinkable through the work of Pierre Bourdieu, whose 'theoretical and methodological toolbox still provides the best way forward for understanding contemporary inequality in terms of its production, reproduction and, importantly, the experience of it'. Threadgold (2011, p. 388) went on to argue that from this perspective 'individual reflexivity can be understood as cultural capital: like language, everyone is using it, but some have the skills and resources to use it better than others'. In this sense young people 'can be as reflexive as possible, but if they cannot put their choices into action, reflexivity becomes an intrinsic part of the reflexive experience of inequality'. For Threadgold (ibid.), agency, the sense and experience of a capacity, an ability 'to put one's choices into practice, or not, can produce a whole gamut of emotions and feelings from confidence, joy and satisfaction to frustration, alienation and withdrawal'.[4]

Our concerns here are less with the theoretical dimensions of this debate – people will continue to locate themselves more or less reflexively in particular systems of thought – and more with the methodological, empirical and even ontological dimensions of youth studies that emerge in these debates. By ontological we mean, for example, is there some sort of experience or feeling or understanding of the realities we encounter and construct that can be defined as a working-class habitus, or an individualised modernity, or a neo-liberal governmentality? As youth studies academics we might want to assemble the social in these or other ways. But does that make them true? Or do we make them true in these ways?

These largely rhetorical questions open a reference to the work of Bruno Latour (2007) in *Reassembling the Social*. The first half of Latour's book is organised around what he calls five major uncertainties: (1) 'the nature of groups: there exist many contradictory ways for actors to be given an identity'; (2) 'the nature of actions: in each course of action a great variety of agents seem to barge in and displace the original goals'; (3) 'the nature of objects: the type of agencies participating in interaction seems to remain wide open'; (4) 'the nature of facts: the links of natural sciences with the rest of society seems to be the source of continuous debates'; (5) '... about the types of studies done under the label of a science of the social as it is never clear in which sense social science can be said to be empirical' (Latour 2007, p. 22).

Latour (ibid.) names these as uncertainties – with a self-acknowledged *weak allusion* to the *uncertainty principle* – because it 'remains impossible to decide whether' the uncertainty 'resides in the observer or in the phenomenon observed'. Latour (2007, p. 43) argues that what he sees as a second source of uncertainty is a fundamental concern that resides at the heart of all the social sciences, namely that action is not *transparent*, and that we need to remain open to the uncertainties at the heart of questions such as: 'When we act, who else is acting? How many agents are also present? How come I never do what I want? Why are we held by forces that are not of our own making?' In an evocative series of gestures he suggests that these uncertainties have troubled the social sciences 'since the time when crowds, masses, statistical norms, invisible hands, and unconscious drives began to replace the passions and reasons, not to mention the angels and demons that had pushed and pulled our humble souls up to then' (ibid.).

Acknowledging this uncertainty does not mean, suggests Latour (2007, p. 50), 'that we should abstain from alluding to hidden variables forever, or that we have to believe that actors live the pristine clarity of some *ego cogito* in full command of their own actions'. Indeed, from Latour's (ibid.) perspective, in which he, and others in the field of actor-network theory, painstakingly disassemble what we think we know of the social and who or what is an *actant* in an array of fields, relationships, assemblages, the 'most powerful insight of social sciences is that other agencies over which we have no control make us do things ... action is distributed among agents, very few of whom look like humans'.

However, what tends to happen in the doing of such things as sociologies of youth, or youth work, or health promotion, a doing often framed by words and concepts such as *society, power, structure* and *context*, is that we 'jump straight ahead to connect vast arrays of life and history, to mobilize gigantic forces, to detect dramatic patterns emerging out of confusing interactions, to see everywhere in the cases at hand yet more examples of well-known types' (Latour 2007, p. 22). The issue here is the movement to put into play pre-existing assumptions about groups, actions, objects, facts and methods, and to force these presumptions to do the work of description, analysis and prediction that they may not be that well suited to. One of the lessons from Latour is that we shouldn't substitute our own certainties or uncertainties for the certainties or uncertainties of other actors. Particularly when we do youth studies and in this doing we seek to make some sense of young people by invoking notions of agency and structure.

So, on the back of this brief sketch of a number of the uncertainties that should be acknowledged in the doing of youth studies, we want to consider some of the limits and possibilities for observing and cataloguing young people's lives and then explaining or making sense of those lives. What is it that we can say about young people, their lives, the things that give particular shape to these lives from the data, even evidence that we might gather from the surveys, the questionnaires, the observations, the interviews, the artefacts that young people might produce if we offer them an opportunity? Particularly if, as is the case in the debate between Woodman and Roberts and Threadgold, a key sociological concern is with ideas of choice and reflexivity and the ways in which 'structures', or 'class', or 'gender', or 'ethnicity', or, even, 'habitus' are imagined as endowing different young people with different capacities for imagining possibilities and exercising choice.

When young people encounter and are represented by sociologists, what often emerges – at least in the published accounts of these encounters in which questions of choice and agency are said to be important – is an overwhelming sense of the young person as a more or less rational being, devoid of emotions or ambivalence. Pain, hurt, hunger, despair, anxiety, decisiveness, uncertainty, ambiguity, irony, humour, longing, desire, loneliness, companionship, love. If we want to we can say that many of these things shape and enable choice or agency. Though these things might be of interest to youth studies, they are not matters, solely, of sociological concepts such as class or individualisation or habitus or reflexivity. Such things can readily be experienced or felt or considered without recourse to any of these concepts, or to the wider institutionalised systems of thought from which they emerge and to which they give shape.

Many of these elements of a life are hard to put into words. Yet it is the words, the inscriptions and marks made by young people that are made to stand in for the complexity and ambivalence that must mark any of our lives, and the passions and drives, the aspirations and reflections, the angels and demons that shape a life and might provide some explanation of a life. As we have argued elsewhere (Kelly 2011), and earlier, when we do social science we too often become literalists: we take what someone says, or the marks that they make, too literally. This literalism accompanies a sense that when we engage with young people we are doing science, gathering data and evidence.

And it is assumed that we can then make what this data means self-evident through the concepts we deploy.

To finish then, we would argue that working with some or all of the following can contribute to discussions that might unsettle the doing of a youth studies (including health promotion with young people) in which the structure–agency debate is unlikely to fade away, even though its contours might shift and change over time and in different spaces.

In the first instance, Foucault's ways of thinking about technologies and practices of the self can unsettle the ways in which we think about agency and structure. For Foucault, technologies and practices of the self emerge in diverse fields of possibilities that are structured by different forms and relations of power that constrain and/or enable young people's life chances, life choices, life courses. So, we might identify and analyse the particular, even more general character of fields of possibilities – classrooms and education systems, workplaces and labour markets, music venues and culture industries – and the relationships between such things as class, status, tastes, gender, sexuality, ability, disability, and the forms of personhood that are encouraged, demanded, allowed in these spaces. The analysis here might be of the less 'principled', more genealogical type suggested by Hunter (1993, 1994). A type that is less concerned with assembling a sense of what agency is, exactly, and what agency is not, and is more concerned with the consequences and outcomes, the choices and responsibilities that become attached to certain ways of being a person in particular, always limited, but never completely closed fields of possibility. As Foucault (1983) argued, freedom does not disappear with the exercise of power. Indeed relations of power are fundamental to the always limited exercise of freedom: a society without power relations must be an abstraction.

In the second instance we might acknowledge, drawing on Zygmunt Bauman's (1989, 1990, 1991) work, that our lives are fundamentally shaped by ambivalence – the very idea of choice and risk makes no sense otherwise – and that there are dangers in doing a social science that tries to *exterminate* that ambivalence. The challenges here are many, but some are both empirical and representational in the sense that we might consider the limits and possibilities of attaching a certain *authenticity* to behaviours, actions or words because they were uttered or acted by a young person; or of claiming a certain *veracity* for the status of marks, inscriptions, words, data because we construct them/it as being objective, or from large scale, statistically valid sets, or from qualitative interviews.

These provocations – and others not included here – need not be imagined as being commensurable with each other. For these things to be useful or productive they don't have to fit together or be amenable to any sort of synthesis. We can instead recognise and work with the limits and possibilities of each, and the tensions that emerge in/between each and the other (Campbell and Kelly 2013). This is something that we have tried to do with our phenomenologically flavoured account of the shifting, always complex relations between what we can identify and locate as the present, the manifestly absent and absent as

Other in Fit to Drive. The middle ground here may appear logical. Even a little safe. What Julia Coffey and David Farrugia (2014) might call 'orthodox'. And this middle ground might produce important understandings of the agency–structure couplet. However, the challenges, as we see them, are to test the limits and possibilities of this couplet, to re-imagine that which we make present, manifestly absent, absent as Other as we take up the opportunities and openings that the work of Foucault, or Bauman, or Latour offers. As Latour (2007, p. 45) argues, if the social sciences are to be revitalised it is 'crucial not to conflate all the agencies overtaking the action into some kind of agency – "society", "culture", "structure", "fields", "individuals", or whatever name they are given – that would itself be social. Action should remain a surprise, a mediation, an event.' It is in this sense that we

> should begin ... not from the 'determination of action by society', the 'calculative abilities of individuals', or the 'power of the unconscious' ... but rather from the under-determination of action, from the uncertainties and controversies about who and what is acting when 'we' act.
>
> (Ibid.)

To finish then, with a gesture towards how these ideas may unsettle, trouble how we understand attempts to encourage young people's agency, understand attempts to encourage 'right thinking' in health promotion programs that are structured by a sense of what is 'good', Latour (2007, p. 46) suggests that we imagine that an 'actor' in the 'hyphenated expression actor-network is not the source of an action but the moving target of a vast array of entities swarming towards it'. In this sense, action is 'borrowed, distributed, suggested, influenced, dominated, betrayed, translated. If an actor is said to be an actor-network, it is first of all to underline that it represents the major source of uncertainty about the origin of action'.

The challenges and opportunities, the limits and possibilities of/for health promotion with young people, and the analysis and critique of health promotion programs that target young people, are fundamentally shaped by what should remain as the uncertainty of that thing we call agency, young people's agency. And by the uncertainties of whatever is that we make present, manifestly absent, absent as Other to agency. The *non-agencies* that shape the capabilities and the capacities of young people to think, to imagine, to do, to act, to be.

Notes

1 With due acknowledgment to Robert Castel (1991), 'From Dangerousness to Risk'. A number of the issues in this section were first canvassed in Kelly 2001.
2 Small bottles – 330–375 ml – of beer in Australia.
3 This section draws, in part, on arguments first presented in Kelly 2014.
4 The exchange has had another instalment from Steven Roberts (2012), but an account of this most recent contribution would add little to what we want to discuss here.

Conclusion

Death and devastation as allegory

The figure of John Law has been a significant presence in this book. Donna Haraway (2008, p. 4) has argued that we can, all of us, be understood as figures, as material-semiotic nodes or knots:

> Figures are not representations or didactic illustrations, but rather material-semiotic nodes or knots in which diverse bodies and meanings coshape one another. For me, figures have always been where the biological and literary or artistic come together with all of the force of the lived reality. My body itself is just such a figure, literally.

So, John Law is a figure who opens us up to an array of methodological conversations. A figure who embodies many of the conversations about knowledge practices in the social sciences that feminists, post-structuralists, actor-network theorists, post-humanists and others have been engaged in during the last 30 or so years. The figure of John Law enables us to open spaces in which we can identify and then discuss the unstable bundling of the array of things that are made present, manifestly absent, and absent as Other in Fit to Drive, and in diverse school based health promotion programs with young people. In these spaces we can imagine what happens when we make the embodied, the aesthetic present in ways that might trouble the limits and possibilities of reason, risk and rationality in such programs. We will come to a final discussion of some of these limits and possibilities shortly. But first, John Law has one final, challenging contribution to make to the work of troubling how it is that we can know … anything.

This contribution emerges from his discussion of how it is that we can know about the horrific deaths and utter devastation of a head-on collision between a Thames Trains commuter train (the '165'), and a First Great Western High Speed Train ('HST') at Ladbroke Grove, just short of London's Paddington rail station, on 5 October 1999. A collision in which thirty-one people died and 400 plus people were injured. As we hope to make apparent, there is much in Law's account of this horrific accident, and what we can know about its causes and consequences, that resonates with our discussions of the ways in which Fit to Drive seeks to impose some order, some reason and rationality, in the wake of the tragic individual and community consequences that are set in chaotic motion by road accidents involving young people.

On that day in October 1999 the 165 and the HST slammed head-on into each other at a closing speed of nearly 250 km per hour. In the subsequent devastation of twisted metal and burnt out carriages the drivers of the two trains and twenty-nine of the 575 passengers aboard both trains were killed. As is the case in the aftermath of horrific incidents of this scale, of this magnitude, there were community, media and political demands to know what happened, what had gone wrong, what had caused the two trains to smash head-on into each other with the death and injury of so many people going about the ordinariness of their commuting and working lives. The subsequent official inquiry, as Law (2004, p. 94), indicates, was charged with identifying and examining 'not only the proximate causes of the accident, but also background factors'.

And it is in this space of needing to know and understand how and why a tragedy such as this was able to happen, the 'proximate causes' and 'background factors' that led to this disaster, that Law proposes two ways of apprehending the Ladbroke Grove accident. For Law (ibid.) the disaster 'can be understood as a bundle of relations and entities'. A number of these are 'brought into presence in the terrible scene of the accident itself'. Still others are 'made manifest as in the form of a context', made 'relevant to that presence in one way or another'. And, finally, others are 'rendered invisible, Othered'. In these ways 'the accident is an object'. In framing the accident as an object Law wants us to think how an accident such as this, a scene of horrific devastation, can also be 'allegorical'.

As we argued in our earlier discussion of Tim Winton's (2008) novel *Breath*, the allegorical can be a powerful and troubling way to think about an array of things, including a sense of self, of place, of time, of human failings, limits and possibilities. In the context of Ladbroke Grove allegory 'does not take the form of statements about reality', but 'if we read between the lines of the carnage it indirectly depicts, enacts and manifests a range of realities'. But, in ways that are different to more direct modes of representation, 'what is made present does not pretend to speak for itself. It calls for interpretation. It presses us into allegory' (Law 2004, p. 94).

These claims also reference ideas that we introduced from Law in our discussion of *Breath*, including a sense that all forms of representation are allegorical. Though claims of direct representation, of factual and evidence-based representations, are allegorical in ways that seek to deny their allegorical nature (Law 2004, pp. 88–89). So, the report of the public inquiry into Ladbroke Grove, charged as it was with having to 'inquire into and draw lessons from the accident … taking account of the findings of … investigations into immediate causes (Law 2004, p. 96, citing the terms of reference for the Inquiry), must conform to various expectations about the gathering of evidence; the review of procedures, protocols and processes; the questioning of staff, of passengers, of witnesses; and the representations of these in the form of a single discursive account of 'proximate causes' and 'background factors'. Even if, as Law (2004, p. 94) argues, this single discursive account can, even should, encounter and interrogate complexities and multiplicities, the 'relations bundled together and brought into presence in the collision'. In this context the possibilities that driver error; or driver recruitment and training; or signalling technologies and/or fault; or the privatised and subcontracted relations between rail operator, railway track owners, and track and signal maintenance companies that may create dangerous, deadly, cracks in what should be a coherent assemblage, are all 'entertained, examined and assessed – and in the report they are accepted or rejected' (Law 2004, p. 96).

In this discussion Law (ibid.) is concerned with the limits and possibilities of knowing that are built into this form of representational, *ontological politics.* As he argues, the 'framing assumptions of Euro-American metaphysics are still hard at work' in the making of the official Inquiry's report, so that a 'coherent account of the world is still possible even at moments when things have gone dreadfully wrong'. The Inquiry, which is 'necessarily allegorical because nothing speaks for itself, nothing is transparent, everything has to be read as a symptom, as being about something else', works to enact presence, manifest absence and absence as Otherness in ways that craft coherence out of chaos.

Troublingly, in ways that Law (2004, p. 97) acknowledges are sometimes too 'dreadful to play with', there is another ontological politics available here, one that is more directly allegorical. In this alternative ontology the Ladbroke Grove accident can be imagined as a 'moment, a dreadful enactment of presence written not in texts and statements, but in steel and flesh and fuel and fire'. Understood in these terms meaning is inscribed, is enacted, as 'impact, collapse, inferno, agonizing pain, terrible burns, grief, panic and death' (Law 2004, p. 96).

The ways of knowing here are more immediately embodied, more visceral, more emotional, even more aesthetic, if aesthetic is not just about beauty. And these ways of knowing have their own limits and possibility. As Law (2004, pp. 96–97) argues, if we engage with the collision as allegory, then we can engage the accident as an 'inscription device that writes its texts not with pens on sheets of paper, but rather with the instruments of kinetic force and fire upon the bodies of people, and the twisted wreckage of gutted rolling stock'. In this way the event 'inscribes itself in and through a theatre of cruelty'.

As an event that demands interpretation, that presses us into allegory, the Ladbroke Grove accident 'crafts and depicts the non-coherence that produced it, the ramifications of a messy organisational and technical hinterland'. Indeed, the collision 'refracts this non-coherence … condenses or articulates it. Terribly, in the bodies, the injuries, and the wreckage. Pain, let us allow, is indeed a witness' (Law 2004, p. 97). But pain is not a witness to a single reality, or to a coherence that we might like to impose after the event. Pain and hurt and loss are in many respects incoherent. We never quite know where they will take us. Where they will leave us. What 'good' they serve. If at all. They are always ambiguous. Open-ended. Troubling to a sense of self. Of others. Of going on. Particularly in cultural formations where we apparently crave *closure*.

What is at stake, then, in making these moves? Certainly not the deliberate, even 'playful' construction of horror, hurt and pain. For Law, what is at stake is how to think about such events, other events, any event. And what to do when such events occur. As he indicates, the representational, ontological politics, and logics and forms, of official inquiries and reports, are one possible move. They are often the only move in contexts where particular, always limited, views of evidence based inquiry and policy development dominate. And this is not a bad thing. But it might be useful to acknowledge that such a move has particular limits to/of/for understanding built into its forms.

Another move is in the direction that Law gestures towards, one that we have been taking at various moments throughout this book. This move towards the embodied, the aesthetic dimensions of meaning making is not about the displacement of representation, of evidence, of reason, risk and rationality. Rather, it has been about what happens to what we know, how we know, if we rub up against the limits and possibilities of reason, risk and rationality. What happens in the act, the process, the practice of troubling or unsettling these limits and possibilities? What happens, what is possible, in this troubling, this unsettling in the particular limits and possibilities of school based health promotion with young people?

Reordering health promotion with young people

Fit to Drive is a highly structured, meticulously choreographed, heavily scripted, continually edited school based intervention into the chaos, incoherence, pain, hurt, suffering and loss that unfolds and engulfs individuals, families, schools and communities in the wake of the death and injury of young people in road accidents. An intervention that tells tragic stories about these accidents. Tragedies that are populated with characters we know too well. Like ourselves. Our brothers and sisters. Our sons and daughters. Our friends. Characters that are human, all too human. Flawed. Prone to hubris. To mistakes. Misjudgements. To overestimating our ability. Underestimating the conditions we find ourselves in. But also, in the moment, oblivious to the possibilities of harm, hurt, danger that become all too apparent after the event. With the luxury of hindsight.

In many respects the tightly structured intervention seeks to impose a coherence after the event. Requires that young people, with guidance, in settings that value their use of a particular style of thought, a particular form of voice, move from this chaos, this incoherence. Move towards ways of knowing that, it is promised, have the capacity, through the development and deployment of facilities for reason and rationality, to fashion, to craft some order from disorder. To put into play evidence, statistics, reason, rationality, even values and morals, in the flight from the chaos and incoherence, the waste and tragedy of young people dying and being hurt in road accidents.

In making these moves we hope, also, to open up spaces in which others might reorder the knowledge practices that take health promotion with young people, in schools and elsewhere, as their object. This reordering, in terms of practice and process and outcomes, should not be prescribed in advance. Should not be proscribed for a number of reasons. For example, we have tried to take seriously how we might approach a description and analysis of a health promotion intervention with young people if we want to trouble and unsettle what is present, what is manifestly absent, what is absent as Other in such programs. So, if in one of our interludes, one of our asides, we engage with a Futurist, Fascist aesthetic that sees beauty, power and erotics in the car-machine-human assemblage we do so not to celebrate this aesthetic. Or to suggest that health promotion with young people should engage with and celebrate such an aesthetic. Rather, our purpose is to imagine some of the elements – speed, beauty, erotics, power – of the hinterland from which Fit to Drive emerges. Elements that are both manifestly absent and absent as Other in the Fit to Drive assemblage. Manifestly absent and absent as Other from a school based health promotion program for young people. In making speed, beauty, erotics and power present in the car-machine-human assemblage we move to a more embodied, allegorical space in which some of the attractions of speed, beauty, erotics and power become apparent. And in becoming apparent the aesthetics of speed, beauty, erotics and power unsettle and trouble the limits and possibilities of reason, risk and rationality in health promotion with young people.

We have tried, also, to take seriously what complexity, multiplicity, ambivalence and ambiguity mean in assembling a health promotion program such as Fit to Drive. And what, as a result, complexity, multiplicity, ambivalence and ambiguity mean in trying to make sense of a program such as Fit to Drive. So, we engaged in some detail with a story about growing up, of being young and male or female in the remote isolation of coastal, rural Western Australia. A story that is about opening yourself and others to the possibility of the harm and danger and excitement to be found in big wave surfing, drug use and fetishistic sexuality. A tale about the risks to be found, the risks to be stumbled upon, in confronting the sheer banality of drawing breath. A story about brushing up against the imagined limits and possibilities of being ordinary. Again, this engagement with an allegorical tale of the horrors, for some young people, of being ordinary should not be read as a celebration of what Foucault might call *limit experiences*. Should not be read as an endorsement of the danger, harm, excitement that Pikelet, Looney, Eva and Sando seek out and embrace. Should not be read as an endorsement of seeking out danger, harm and excitement so as not to be ordinary. Recklessness, if this is what it is, is not what we sought to make present here. Instead, what we wanted to explore was what might emerge, become apparent, beyond practices of reason and rationality when some people, young or old, do *dumb* things, do dangerous things, do risky things. If we can imagine that danger, harm and excitement are experienced and felt and engaged with differently, at different times, in different contexts, by different individuals and groups, then we must acknowledge that choice and risks *only* make sense in contexts, spaces and relationships that are always ambivalent and ambiguous, always complex and multiple. The challenge, as we see it, in working with a social science of risk, a social science of young people and risk, is not to exterminate that ambivalence (Kelly 2014).

We have, further, tried to take seriously what an extensive and detailed engagement with the embodied, the aesthetic, means for trying to understand the ways in which young people make some sense of the stories, the logics, the practices and activities that give form to something such as Fit to Drive. And in this move we have tried to engage with the problem of death. An engagement structured through a sense that not all deaths are tragic. That there might be, can be, something like a *good* death. Again, the moves we made in this direction should not be read as signalling, somehow, that we are trivialising the deaths of young people in road accidents; that we are making some claim that health promotion with young people should necessarily imagine that the deaths of young people, the lives cut short, the possibility and potential erased, loss and pain and hurt, are less than tragic, are something other than tragic. That would be, to understate by some order of magnitude, insensitive. What we wanted to do was suggest that a posthuman theory of death opens up the problem of death to the problem of life. Without one the other makes no sense. Cannot be. And in making this move we unsettle a one dimensional view of death, of life. Complexity, multiplicity, ambivalence and ambiguity are then no longer absent from the problem of death, the problem of life.

So, does a young person's death look and feel the same for a middle aged school principal, or a grieving parent who can imagine a life of promise and possibility, or for a young person's peers who might imagine death as being about release, or an end to pain, an end to anguish, or as being made glamorous in ways that attach an attractiveness to its possibility? Indeed, this possibility is something that is made present, widely, often, in music, in film, in literature in ways that just don't seem possible for school based health promotion. In Julian Barnes' (2011, pp. 12–14) acclaimed novel, *The Sense of an Ending*, his main characters, the then school-aged young men Tony Webster, Adrian Finn, Alex and Colin, speak to the trope of a young death that is seen as heroic, glamourous, even attractive, in ways that may disturb many adults. The young men, in this telling, participate in a Monday morning school assembly at an English grammar school in the early 1960s, where their headmaster, with much gravity and solemnity, informs them that one of their fellow pupils, Robson of the Science Sixth (form), had died over the weekend. The headmaster made much of the tragedy of a life cut short, of what Robson's death meant as loss to the school. But Tony and Adrian and Alex and Colin didn't imagine, or make sense of Robson's death in these terms, in terms of tragedy. For them mystery, glamour, envy and notoriety came rushing into the space opened by his death.

More so, as we come to know, after they discovered that Robson had committed suicide when he found out that he had made his girlfriend pregnant. And these non-tragic dimensions of a young death made themselves felt in ways that provoked some disdain. Robson, for these young men, didn't embody the imagination, the philosophical seriousness they deemed as necessary accompaniments to the *ethical* and *aesthetic* questions associated with the act of taking one's own life.

And, finally, we have made these moves to unsettle the ways in which dominant discourses of risk are never just about the evidence based calculation and categorisation of possibilities and probabilities. Are never just about the likely future consequences of an array of pasts and presents. Though they will be about these. Risk and danger, harm and hurt, as they are imagined in many of the discourses that inform school based health promotion interventions with young people, emerge from hinterlands in which individualised responsibilities for the management and promotion of physical and mental health and well-being go hand-in-hand with a sense that these responsibilities emerge in the practice of choices, good and bad. We have sought to unsettle some of these powerful ideas about choices and responsibilities, about young people's voice and their agency. Not, as some might say, to deny the possibility of choice and agency if those things are imagined as important, as a good. We all have choices to make, large and small, consequential and not so much. Instead, we have wanted to explore the limits and possibilities of the *idea* and the practice of choice and agency. To trouble the investments that youth studies, youth work, school based health promotion with young people have in particular, always limited, views of voice and agency, of right-thinking. We wanted to unsettle the moral and value-laden dimensions of choice and agency when these are deployed and operationalised in practices such as small group problem solving, or values clarification sessions and workshops. When, in this deployment and operationalisation, choice, agency, values and morals are often enclosed, often encounter enclosure, in the particular *irreality* of school based health promotion interventions with young people. What possibilities, practices and processes emerge on the horizons of these spaces if we acknowledge the complexity, the ambivalence, the ambiguity that always shapes any examination, any exploration of choices, responsibilities, values and morals?

In troubling and reordering health promotion with young people, and the description, discussion, analysis and critique of health promotion with young people, we ask an array of questions about how it is that we can know something, can know anything. But undecidability is not the only possibility. We are always confronted with other possibilities. And in doing and discussing health promotion with young people, one of these possibilities is to ask, *What can we do?* In recognising this imperative to ask *What can we do?* we acknowledge that in wanting to do something we look to the possibility and promise of meaning and coherence in the face of chaos and hurt and harm and risk. In the face of incoherence. In this recognition we can ask what is lost, what is made absent, when we force coherence on incoherence. And we must ask what we gain, what we make present, when we craft and assemble coherence in the face of the apparently incoherent, the undecidable. Here, once again, John Law provides a final contribution to understanding some of limits and possibilities in the myriad encounters, the ongoing dance between coherence and incoherence. This contribution emerges from his concern with the binary dimensions, the 'coherence' that is forced on the relations between the coherent, the non-coherent. For Law (2004, p. 100) the concept of gathering, its relation to ideas of crafting and bundling, is more suggestive of what is possible if we think of assemblages as being loosely coupled, as being emergent. Gathering, here (see also Kamp and Kelly 2014), speaks to practices, ways of knowing, enactments that can be made in answer to *What can we do?*

> To gather is to bring 'to-gether'. To relate. To pick (as with a bunch of flowers). To meet together. To flow together ... To build up or add to (as with a gathering storm, or gathering darkness ...). Gathering, then, has its own connotations. But it tells us nothing of consistency or inconsistency. And nothing of coherence, incoherence or non-coherence. Here, then, it is symmetrical.

Our final Interlude, which may, indeed, be more Aesop than Aeschylus, gestures to the goods that can emerge in the more prosaic dimensions of everyday assemblages, everyday *gatherings.* This Interlude speaks, as allegory, to things such as 'community', 'educating for the Good', 'intergenerational relations and practices', 'care', responsibility', 'obligation', ... *What can we do?* must remain a question that requires us to craft and make things present, manifestly absent, absent as Other. With questions about truth, politics, justice, spirituality, aesthetics, among an array of possibilities, always in play. But in play in ways that shouldn't be determined in advance. Because *What can we do?* may well be an inescapable, and always ambivalent, dimension of what it means to be human, all too human.

Interlude: Kerry's story

The boy was, I would guess, about 10 or 11. All gangly limbs. Ears prominent below his helmet. A few brown curls growing out of his new school year haircut. Perched on a seat that looked too high for him, precariously leaning over to the left, toes just reaching the ground in an effort to hold his bike steady, he was looking intently, almost apprehensively, to the right and left, and back again, as the trickle of cars passed in front of him.

I had pulled up behind him where the Upfield rail-line bike path crossed Hope Street, in Brunswick, an inner-city suburb of Melbourne, Australia. It wasn't one of the trickier intersections, such as Albion Street, where the path slopes down to a busy feeder road, with steady streams of pedestrians making a bee-line for Anstey railway station on the other side, and where you're just as likely to encounter a bus idling at the bus stop, blocking your path and your line of vision across the road. Hope Street, by contrast, feels very much like it did when I first started doing the ride from Coburg to work in the city over twenty years ago. Along the stretch of road between the railway line and Sydney Road, the light industry and small warehouses are reminders of the bustling industry base of the suburb of the past. Now, however, there are few workers making their way to those modest factories and workshops, and the street itself is relatively quiet this time of morning.

It was earlier than my usual riding time, and there weren't many riders on the bike track. I was glad of this. Relieved the boy would be spared the additional pressure of impatient riders shooting past him as he waited until he felt safe enough to cross. Ten year old boys learning to ride a bike are simultaneously observing what other riders are doing. They notice the young men in their twenties, costumed, and riding as if they were competing in the Giro D'Italia. Whipping in and out of the lane. Narrowly missing riders coming in the opposite direction. Women with strollers, school children and couples walking their dogs. Young children waiting with other riders at the intersections take note that many cyclists don't wait for lights to change before darting across. They get startled, as they're about to take off, by the cyclist who dashes past them hardly pausing to properly check that the road is clear. In Melbourne, commuting by bike has become for many, it seems, as earnest and frantic, as competitive, as modern life.

Pulling up a metre or so behind the boy to allow him some space until he judged it safe to cross, I looked behind me. There were a couple of riders lined up along the path, muffled against the morning chill in scarves and gloves, waiting with an air of patient detachment for the line to get moving. We followed the boy at a leisurely pace for a kilometre, stopping for lights, or traffic, at half a dozen crossroads along the way. At Dawson St, still immediately behind him, I looked back again. Our conga line of morning commuters had increased to a dozen or more riders. Miraculously, none had attempted to pass, to harry or harass the boy, even unintentionally, by forming a drag race starting pack beside him at the lights. All still seemed content to allow the boy to set the pace.

References

Abbott-Chapman, J, Denhom, C and Wyld, C 2008, 'Social support as a factor inhibiting teenage risk-taking: views of students, parents and professionals', *Journal of Youth Studies*, vol. 11, no. 6, pp. 611–627.

Abel, T 2007, 'Cultural capital in health promotion', in D V McQueen and I Kickbusch (eds), *Health and modernity: the role of theory in health promotion*, Springer, New York.

Aesop, 2008, *Aesop's fables: translated with an introduction and notes by Laura Gibbs*, Oxford University Press, Oxford and New York.

Ariens, B 2007, *Facilitator training notes*, f2d, Melbourne.

Ariens, B 2010, *F2D (Fit to Drive) facilitator script and manual*, f2d, Melbourne.

Arnett, J J 1996, 'Sensation seeking, aggressiveness, and adolescent reckless behavior', *Personality and individual differences*, no. 20, pp. 693–702.

'Arrive Alive, Victoria's road safety strategy 2012', www.roadsafety.vic.gov.au/about/about_the_arrive_alive_strategy.html

Austen, J 1996, *Pride and prejudice*, Penguin, London.

Australian Institute of Health and Welfare 2007, *Young Australians: their health and wellbeing*, Australian Institute of Health and Welfare, Canberra.

Australian Institute of Health and Welfare 2011, *Young Australians: their health and wellbeing 2011*, Australian Institute of Health and Welfare, Canberra.

Australian Transport Council 2011, 'National road safety strategy 2011–2020', viewed 8 August 2012, www.atcouncil.gov.au/documents/files/NRSS_2011_2020_15Aug11pdf

Australian Transport Safety Bureau 2004, *Young people and road crashes*, Australian Government, Canberra ACT.

Bakhtin, M 1981, *The dialogic imagination: four essays*, University of Texas Press, Austin.

Balbo, L 2007, 'Thinking health promotion sociologically', in D V McQueen and I Kickbusch (eds), *Health and modernity: the role of theory in health promotion*, Springer, New York.

Barnes, J 2011, *The sense of an ending*, Jonathan Cape, London.

Batsleer, J 2008, *Informal learning in youth work*, Sage, Los Angeles and London.

Batsleer, J and Davies, B (eds) 2010, *What is youth work?*, Learning Matters, Exeter.

Bauman, Z 1989, *Modernity and the holocaust*, Polity Press, Cambridge.

Bauman, Z 1990, 'Modernity and ambivalence', in M. Featherstone (ed.), *Global culture*, Sage, London, pp. 143–170.

Bauman, Z 1991, *Modernity and ambivalence*, Polity Press, Cambridge.

Bauman, Z 2008, *Does ethics have a chance in a world of consumers?* Harvard University Press, Cambridge MA.

Beck, U 1992, *Risk society: towards a new modernity*, Sage, London.

Beck, U 1999, *World risk society*, Polity Press, Cambridge.

Beck-Gernsheim, E 2000, 'Health and Responsibility: From Social Change to Technologica; Change and Vice Versa' in A Adam, U Beck and J Van Loon (eds), *The risk society and beyond: critical issues for social theory*, Sage, London.

Begley, S 2000, 'Getting inside a teen brain', *Newsweek*, vol. 135, no. 9, pp. 58–59.

Benjamin, J and Rabinach, A 1996, 'Foreword', in K Theweleit, *Male fantasies volume 2. Male bodies: psychanalysing the white terror*, University of Minnesota Press, Minneapolis.

Bennett, D 2007, 'Adolescent development and risk-taking', viewed 10 July 2009, www.yapa.org.au/youth/facts/devriskphp

Bernstein, M 1994, *Foregone conclusions: against apocalyptic history*, University of California Press, Berkeley.

Bessant, J 2002, 'Generative metaphor, problem setting in policy and the discovery of youth at risk', *Youth and Policy: The Journal of Critical Analysis, UK*, no. 76, pp. 33–46.

Bessant, J 2008, 'Hard wired for risk: neurological science, "the adolescent brain" and developmental theory', *Journal of Youth Studies*, vol. 11, no. 3, pp. 349–362.

Bessant, J 2009, 'Aristotle meets youth work: a case for virtue ethics', *Journal of Youth Studies*, vol. 12, no. 4, pp. 425–440.

Bessant, J, Hill, R and Watts, R 2003, *'Discovering' risk: social research and policy making*, Peter Lang, New York.

Bessant, J, Sercombe, H and Watts, R 1998, *Youth studies: an Australian perspective*, Pearson, Melbourne.

Best, A 2006, *Fast cars, cool rides: the accelerating world of young people and their cars*, New York Press, New York.

Best, A 2008, 'Teen driving as public drama: statistics, risk, and the social construction of youth as a public problem', *Journal of Youth Studies*, vol. 11, no. 6, pp. 661–669.

Biddulph, S 2007, 'Mentally, teens drive best alone', *Sydney Morning Herald*, 11 January.

Bina, M, Graziano, F and Bonino, S 2006, 'Risky driving and lifestyles in adolescence', *Accident Analysis and Prevention*, vol. 38, pp. 472–481.

Bingham, C R and Shope, J T 2004, 'Adolescent developmental antecedents of risky driving among young adults', *Journal of Studies on Alcohol*, vol. 65, no. 1, pp. 84–94.

Blum, R 1988, 'Adolescent health in a time of change', in D Bennett and M Williams (eds), *New universals: adolescent health in a time of change*, Brolga Press, Melbourne.

Boal, A 2000, *Theatre of the oppressed*, Pluto Press, London.

Bolton, R 1986, *People skills: how to assert yourself, listen to others, and resolve conflicts*, Prentice Hall, Sydney.

Bourdieu, P 1990, *The logic of practice*, Stanford University Press, Stanford.

Braidotti, R. 2013, *The posthuman*, Polity Press, Cambridge.

Brecht, B 1963, *Schriften zum Theater 1. Einmalige Sonderausgabe*, Suhrkamp Verlag, Frankfurt am Main.

Brecht, B 1976, *Poems: Part Two 1929–1938*, ed. J Willett, trans. R Manheim, Eyre Methuen, London.

Brook, P 1996, *The empty space: a book about the theatre: deadly, holy, rough, immediate*, Penguin, London.
Bruner, J 1990, *Acts of meaning*, Harvard University Press, Cambridge MA.
Burchell, G 1996, 'Liberal government and techniques of the self', in A Barry, T Osborne and N Rose (eds) *Foucault and political reason: liberalism, neo-liberalism and rationalities of government*, UCL Press, London, pp. 19–36.
Burley, L 2009, 'Seven teens in horrific car crash', *The Chronicle*, viewed 28 May 2009, www.finda.com.au/story/2009/05/04/seven-teens-in-horrific-car-crash/
Buytendijk, F J J 1973, *Pain*, Greenwood Press, Westport CT.
Campbell, P and Kelly, P 2013, 'In/between feminism and Foucault: Iraqi women's warblogs and intellectual practices of the self', *Critical Sociology*, vol. 39, no. 2, 183–199.
Carmody, M 2009, *Sex and ethics young people and ethical sex*, Palgrave Macmillan, South Yarra, Australia.
Carr-Gregg, M 2007, 'The answers to an accident', *Herald Sun*, 11 December.
Castel, R 1991, 'From dangerousness to risk', in G Burchell, C Gordon, and P Miller (eds), *The Foucault effect: studies in governmental rationality*, Harvester Wheatsheaf, Hemel Hempstead, pp. 281–298.
Catalyst 2005, 'Teen brain', television broadcast, ABC Television, 28 July, www.abc.net.au/catalyst/stories/s1424747htm
Catchpole, J and Styles, T 2005, *Young drivers: who takes risks and why?*Research report ARR 364, ARRB Group, Vermont South, Victoria.
Cavallo, A 1994, 'High-risk behaviours, youth and road accidents: background paper, VicRoads workshop', VicRoads, Kew, Victoria.
Cavallo, A 2004, 'Young driver crashes in Victoria', paper presented at the Saferoads Conference, Melbourne, Victoria, April.
Cavallo, A, Montero, K, Sangster, J and Maunders, D 1997, *Youth work with high risk young drivers: VicRoads and RMIT peer education program*, RMIT, Melbourne.
Cavallo, A and Triggs, T J 1996, *Young driver research strategy report no. 85*, Monash University Accident Research Centre, Melbourne.
Cebulla, A 2009, 'Risk through the years: a statistical portrait of young people's risk perceptions and experiences relative to those of older generations', *Journal of Youth Studies*, vol. 12, no. 1, pp. 39–56.
Chamberlain, C and Mackenzie, D 1998, *Youth homelessness: early intervention and prevention*, Australian Centre for Equity through Education, Sydney.
Clendinnen, I 2005, *Dancing with strangers: Europeans and Australians at first contact*, Cambridge University Press, Cambridge and New York.
Clifford, J 1986, 'On ethnographic allegory', in J. Clifford and G E Marcus (eds), *Writing culture: the poetics and politics of ethnography*, University of California Press, Berkeley CA, pp. 98–121.
Coffey, J and Farrugia, D 2014, 'Unpacking the black box: the problem of agency in the sociology of youth', *Journal of Youth Studies*, vol. 17, no. 4, pp. 461–474.
Collins, R 1984, 'The role of emotion in social structure', in K R Scherer and P Ekman (eds), *Approaches to emotion*, Lawrence Erlbaum, Hillsdale NJ.
Colquhouon, D, Goltz, K and Sheehan, M (eds) 1997, *The health promoting school: policy, programmes and practice in Australia*, Harcourt Brace and Company Australia, New South Wales.
Commonwealth Department of Health and Family Services 2000, *A national framework for health promoting schools (2000–2003)*, Author, Canberra.

Connell, R W 2000, *The men and the boys*, Allen and Unwin, St Leonards, NSW.

Corney, T 2004, 'Values versus competencies: implications for the future of professional youth work education', *Journal of Youth Studies*, vol. 7, no. 4, pp. 513–527.

Corney, T 2006, 'Youth work in schools. Should youth workers also be teachers?' *Youth Studies Australia*, vol. 25, no. 3, pp. 17–25.

Crawshaw, P 2004, 'The "logic of practice" in the risky community: the potential of the work of Pierre Bourdieu for theorising young men's risk-taking', in W Mitchell, R Bunton and E Green (eds), *Young people, risk and leisure: constructing identities in everyday life*, Palgrave Macmillan, Basingstoke.

Crisp, S 2010, 'Learning to take risks is an essential part of growing up', *The Age*, 20 May 2010, viewed 30 May 2010, www.theage.com.au/opinion/society-and-culture/learning-to-take-risks-is-an-essential-part-of-growing-up-20100519-vf38.html#ixzz2Qb55olvp

Crockett, J 2012, '"There's nothing the *@#! wrong with me": youth mental health and substance use in rural and remote Australia and the potential role of school-based interventions', *Youth Studies Australia*, vol. 31 no. 1, pp. 53–59.

Csapo, E 2010, *Actors and icons of the ancient theatre*, Wiley-Blackwell, Chichester.

Csapo, E and Miller, M C (eds) 2007, *The origins of theatre in Ancient Greece and beyond*, Cambridge University Press, Cambridge and New York.

Dahl, R 2008, 'Biological, developmental, and neurobehavioural factors relevant to adolescent driving risks', *American Journal of Preventative Medicine*, vol. 35, pp. 278–284.

Damasio, A 1999, *The feeling of what happens: body and emotion in the making of consciousness*, Harvest, San Diego CA.

Damasio, A 2005, *Descartes' error: emotion, reason and the human brain*, Penguin, London.

Davis, N J 1999, *Youth crisis: growing up in the high-risk society*, Praeger, Westport CT.

DEECD (Department of Education and Early Childhood Development) 2007, 'Student learning initiatives: whole school implementation action plan', viewed 9 November 2009, www.educationvic.gov.au/studentlearning/curriculum/preptoyear10/guidelines/phase2/ws/impactionplanhtm

Denzin, N and Lincoln, Y 2008, *Strategies of qualitative inquiry*, Sage, Thousand Oaks CA.

Dewey, J 1997, *Experience and education*, Touchstone, New York.

Doherty, S T, Andrey, J C and MacGregor, C 1998, 'The situational risks of young drivers: the influence of passengers, time of day and day of week on accident rates', *Accident Analysis and Prevention*, vol. 30, pp. 45–52.

Douglas, M 1992, *Risk and blame: essays in cultural theory*, Routledge, London.

Douglas, T 1991, *A handbook of common groupwork problems*, Tavistock/Routledge, London and New York.

Dutta, S (ed.) 2004, *Greek tragedy*, Penguin, London.

Eckersley, R 1988, *Casualties of change: the predicament of youth in Australia*, Australian Commission for the Future, Melbourne.

Eckersley, R 1992, *Youth and the challenge to change: apocalypse? No!*Essay series no. 1, Australian Commission for the Future, Melbourne.

Eckersley, R 2005, *Well and good: morality, meaning and happiness*, 2nd edn, Text, Melbourne.

Eco, U 2004, *On beauty: a history of a western idea*, MacLehose Press, London.

Eldridge, D 2008, 'Injury among young Australians', *AIHW bulletin no 60*, Cat no. AUS 102, AIHW, Canberra.

Ellis, R 2006, 'Phenomenology-friendly neuroscience: the return to Merleau-Ponty as psychologist', *Human Studies*, vol. 29, no. 1, pp. 33–55.

Ellos, W 1994, *Narrative ethics*, Avebury, Aldershot.

Erikson, E 1971, *Identity: youth and crisis*, Faber and Faber, London.

European Commission n.d., 'Intelligent transport systems mobility and transport', viewed 18 October 2012.

Evans, K 2007, 'Concepts of bounded agency in education, work, and the personal lives of young adults', *International Journal of Psychology*, vol. 42, no. 2, pp. 85–93.

Ewald, F 1991, 'Insurance and risks', in G Burchell, C Gordon and P Miller (eds), *The Foucault effect: studies in governmentality*, University of Chicago Press, Chicago.

Ferguson, S, Teoh, E and McCartt, A T 2007, 'Progress in teenage crash risk during the last decade', *Journal of Safety Research*, vol. 38, no. 2, pp. 137–145.

Fischer-Lichte, E 2005, *Theatre, sacrifice, ritual: exploring forms of political theatre*, Routledge, London and New York.

Flanagan, R 2008, *Wanting*, Knopf, Sydney NSW.

Flanagan, R 2013, *The narrow road to the deep north*, Random House, Sydney NSW.

Flyvbjerg, B 2006, *Making social science matter: why social inquiry fails and how it can succeed again*, Cambridge University Press, Cambridge.

Forster, E M 1987, *A passage to India*, The Great Writers Library, London.

Forster, E M 1989, *Howards End*, Penguin, London.

Foucault, M 1983, 'The subject and power', in H L Dreyfus and P Rabinow (eds), *Michel Foucault: beyond structuralism and hermeneutics*, University of Chicago Press, Chicago.

Foucault, M 1985, *The use of pleasure*, Pantheon, New York.

Foucault, M 1986, *The care of the self*, Pantheon, New York.

Foucault, M 1991, 'Governmentality', in G Burchell, C Gordon and P Miller (eds), *The Foucault effect: studies in governmental rationaltiy*, Harvester Wheatsheaf, Hemel Hempstead, pp. 87–104.

France, A 2000, 'Towards a sociological understanding of youth and their risk-taking', *Journal of Youth Studies*, vol. 3, pp. 317–331.

Franze, M and Paulus, P 2009, 'Mind Matters: a programme for the promotion of mental health in primary and secondary schools', *Health Education*, vol. 109, no. 4, pp. 369–379.

Franzkoviak, P 1988, 'Life in the fast lane: adolescent risk-taking as a major challenge to health promotion', in D Bennett and M Williams (eds), *New universals: adolescent health in a time of change*, Brolga Press, Melbourne.

Furlong, A and Cartmel, F 1997, *Young people and social change: individualisation and risk in late modernity*, Open University Press, Buckingham.

Gadamer, H-G 2006, *Truth and method*, 2nd, revised edn, Continuum, London and New York.

Gaskell, E 2000, *Cranford*, Oxford University Press, Oxford.

Gendlin, E 1962, *Experiencing and the creation of meaning: a philosophical and psychological approach to the subjective*, Free Press of Glencoe, New York.

Gendlin, E T 1991, 'Crossing and dipping: some terms for approaching the interface between natural understanding and logical formulation', in M Galbraith and W J Rapaport (eds), *Subjectivity and the debate over computational cognitive science*, SUNY Press, Buffalo NY.

Gendlin, E 1995, 'Crossing and dipping: some terms for approaching the interface between natural understanding and logical formulation', *Mind and Machines*, vol. 5, pp. 547–560.

Gendlin, E T 1997,'How philosophy cannot appeal to experience, and how it can', in D M Levin (ed.), *Language beyond postmodernism: saying and thinking in Gendlin's philosophy*, Northwestern University Press, Evanston IL.

Gergen, K J and Gergen, M 1983, 'Narratives of the self', in K Scheibe and T Harben (eds), *Studies in social identity*, Praeger, New York.

Giddens, A 1991, *Modernity and self identity*, Polity Press, Cambridge.

Giedd, J N 2004, 'Structural magnetic resonance imaging of the adolescent brain', *Annals of the New York Academy of Sciences*, vol. 1021, pp. 77–85.

Giedd, J N, Blumenthal, J, Jeffries, N O, Castellanos, F X, Liu, H, Zijdenbos, A, Paus, T, Evans, A C and Rapoport, J L 1999, 'Brain development during childhood and adolescence: a longitudinal MRI study', *Nature Neuroscience*, vol. 2, no. 10, pp. 861–863.

Global Road Safety Partnership 2001, 'Road safety education in schools: saving young lives and limbs', viewed 30 April 2008, www.grsproadsafety.org/themes/default/pdfs/Road%20safety%20education%20in%20schoolspdf

Goffman, E 1980, *The presentation of self in everyday life*, Penguin, Harmondsworth.

Gould, S J 1981, *The mismeasure of man*, Norton, New York.

Graham, H and White, R 2007, 'Young people, dangerous driving and car culture', *Youth Studies Australia*, vol. 26, no. 3, pp. 28–35.

Grayling, A C 2007, *What is good? The search for the best way to live*, Phoenix, London.

Grosz, E 1995, *Space, time and perversion, essays on the politics of bodies*, Routledge, New York.

Gubrium, J F and Holstein, J A 2009, *Analyzing narrative reality*, Sage, Thousand Oaks CA.

Gullone, E and Moore, S 2000, 'Adolescent risk-taking and the five factor model of personality', *Journal of Adolescence*, vol. 23, pp. 393–407.

Hall, G S 1931, *Adolescence, its psychology and its relations to physiology, anthropology, sociology sex, crime, religion and education: volume 1*, D Appleton and Co, New York.

Haraway, D 1991, *Simians, cyborgs, and women: the reinvention of nature*, Routledge, New York.

Haraway, D 2008, '"There are always more things going on than you thought!" Methodologies as thinking technologies', in A Smelik and N Lykke (eds), *Bits of life: feminism at the intersection of media, bioscience and technology*, University of Washington Press, Seattle, pp. 32–41.

Harris, A 2004, *Future girl: young women in the twenty-first century*, Routledge, New York and London.

Harrison, L, Kelly, P, Lindsay, J, Advocat, J and Hickey, C 2011, '"I don't know anyone that has two drinks a day": young people, alcohol and the government of pleasure', *Health, Risk and Society*, vol. 13, no. 5, pp. 469–486.

Harrison, W 2006, *Fatigue and young drivers*, RACV, Melbourne.

Hartnoll, P 2003, *The theatre: a concise history*, 3rd edn, Thames and Hudson, New York.

Hatfield, J and Fernandes, R 2009, 'The role of risk-propensity in the risky driving of younger drivers', *Accident Analysis and Prevention* vol. 41, pp. 25–35.

Hawkins, J D, Catalano, R F, Kosterman, R, Abbott, R and Hill, K G 1999, 'Preventing adolescent health-risk behaviours by strengthening protection during childhood', *Archive of Pediatric Adolescent Medicine*, vol. 153, pp. 226–234.
Hawkins, J D, Catalano, R F and Miller, J, 1992, 'Risk and protective factors for alcohol and other drug problems in adolescence and early childhood: implications for substance abuse prevention', *Psychological Bulletin*, vol. 112, pp. 64–105.
Hayles, K 1999, *How we became posthuman: virtual bodies in cybernetics, literature, and informatics*, University of Chicago Press, Chicago.
Hayman, S 2015, 'Shelia Kitzinger obituary', *Guardian*, 12 April, www.theguardian.com/lifeandstyle/2015/apr/12/sheila-kitzinger, accessed 7 July 2015.
Healy, P 1994, 'Rationality, judgment and rule-following: a reply to Reiner', *Electronic Journal of Analytic Philosophy*, vol. 2, no. 4, www.ejap.louisiana.edu/
Healy, D, Catchpole, J and Harrison, W 2012, *Victoria's graduated licensing system evaluation interim report for VicRoads*, Authors, Melbourne.
Hedlund, J, Shults, R A and Compton, R 2003, 'What we know, what we don't know, and what we need to know about graduated driver licensing', *Journal of Safety Research*, vol. 34, no. 1, pp. 107–115.
Herbrechter, S 2013, 'The roar on the other side of silence … or, what's left of the humanities? Review of Rosi Braidotti's *The Posthuman*', *Culture Machine*, April, pp. 1–13.
Hewitt, J, Regoli, R and Kierkus, C A 2006, 'Adolescent risk-taking as a justification for paternalistic legal policy', *Justice Policy Journal*, vol. 3, no. 2, pp. 1–31.
Horvath, C , Lewis, I and Watson, B 2012, 'The beliefs which motivate young male and female drivers to speed: a comparison of low and high intenders', *Accident Analysis and Prevention*, no. 45, pp. 334–341.
Hume, D 2007, *An enquiry concerning human understanding*, Oxford University Press, Oxford and New York.
Hunter, I 1993, 'Subjectivity and government', *Economy and Society*, vol. 22, no. 1, pp. 121–134.
Hunter, I 1994, *Rethinking the school*, St. Martins Press, New York.
Imberger, K, Walsh, K, Catchpole, J and Pyta, V 2011, *Development of advertisements to address risk taking by young drivers*, ARRB Group, viewed 8 September 2012, http://casradelaide.edu.au/rsr/RSR2011/6CPaper%20026%20Imbergerpdf
Ingram, I and Harris, J 2001, *Delivering good youth work: a working guide to surviving and thriving*, Russell House, Lyme Regis.
Ioannou, S, Kouta, C and Charalambous, N 2012, 'Moving from health education to health promotion: developing the health education curriculum in Cyprus', *Health Education*, vol. 112, no. 2, pp. 153–169.
Jain, S 2006, 'Urban violence: luxury in made space', in M Sheller and J Urry (eds), *Mobile technologies of the city*, Routledge, New York and London.
James, W 1890/1950, *The principles of psychology*, Macmillan, London.
James, W 1899, *Talks to teachers on psychology: and to students on some of life's ideals*, Longmans, Green, London.
James, W 2010, *The heart of William James: edited and with an introduction by Robert Richardson*, Harvard University Press, Cambridge MA.
Jarvis, P 2006, *Towards a comprehensive theory of human learning: lifelong learning and the learning society vol. 1*, Routledge, London and New York.
Jessor, R 1987, 'Risky driving and adolescent problem behaviour: an extension of problem-behaviour theory', *Alcohol, Drugs and Driving*, vol. 2, pp. 1–12.

Jessor, R 1991, 'Risk behavior in adolescence: a psychosocial framework for understanding and action', *Journal of Adolescent Health*, vol. 12, pp. 597–605.

Jessor, R and Jessor, J L 1977, *Problem behavior and psychosocial development: a longitudinal study of youth*, Academic Press, New York.

Jessor, R, Turbin, M S and Costa, F M 1997, 'Risk and protection in successful outcomes among disadvantaged adolescents', *Applied Developmental Science*, vol. 2 no. 4, pp. 194–208.

Johnson, M 1987, *Body in the mind: the bodily basis of meaning, imagination and reason*, University of Chicago Press, Chicago.

Johnson, M 2007, *The meaning of the body*, University of Chicago Press, Chicago.

Johnson, D W and Johnson, F P 2003, *Joining together: group theory and group skills*, Allyn and Bacon, Boston.

Jones, G 2009, *Youth*, Polity, Cambridge.

Jong-wook, L 2006, 'Opening address', *Health Promotion International*, vol. 21 no. S1, p. 6.

Kamp, A and Kelly, P 2014, 'Once were young: reflexive hindsight and the problem of teen parents', *Journal of Youth Studies*, vol. 17, no. 7, pp. 887–900.

Katz, J 1999, *How emotions work*, University of Chicago Press, Chicago and London.

Keating, D P and Halpern-Felsher, B L 2008, 'Adolescent drivers: a developmental perspective on risk, proficiency, and safety', *American Journal of Preventive Medicine*, vol. 35, Supplement 1, pp. 272–277.

Kelly, P 1998, 'Risk and the regulation of youth(ful) identities in an age of manufactured uncertainty', Ph.D. thesis, Deakin University.

Kelly, P 1999, 'Wild and tame zones: regulating the transitions of youth at risk', *Journal of Youth Studies*, vol. 2, no. 2, pp. 193–219.

Kelly, P 2001, 'Youth at risk: processes of responsibilization and individualization in the risk society', *Discourse*, vol. 22, no. 1, pp. 23–34.

Kelly, P 2003, 'Growing up as risky business? Risks, surveillance and the institutionalised mistrust of youth', *Journal of Youth Studies*, vol. 6, no. 2, pp. 165–180.

Kelly, P 2006, 'The entrepreneurial self and "youth at risk": exploring the horizons of identity in the twenty-first century', *Journal of Youth Studies*, vol. 9 no. 1, pp. 17–32.

Kelly, P 2007, 'Governing individualized risk biographies: new class intellectuals and the problem of youth at-risk', *British Journal of Sociology of Education*, vol. 28, no. 1, pp. 39–53.

Kelly, P 2011, '*Breath* and the truths of youth at-risk: allegory and the social scientific imagination', *Journal of Youth Studies*, vol. 14, no. 4, pp. 431–447.

Kelly, P 2012, 'The brain in the jar', *Journal of Youth Studies*, vol. 15, no. 7, pp. 944–959.

Kelly, P 2013, *The self as enterprise: Foucault and the 'spirit' of 21st century capitalism*, Ashgate/Gower, Aldershot.

Kelly, P 2014, 'Youth studies and the problem of agency: Foucault vs Marx, Tait vs Sercombe; Beck vs Bourdieu, Woodman vs Threadgold vs Roberts', in S Baker, B Buttigieg and B Robards (eds), *Youth cultures and subcultures*, Ashgate, Aldershot.

Kemshall, H 2008, 'Risks, rights and justice: understanding and responding to youth risk', *Youth Justice*, vol. 8 , no. 1, pp. 21–37.

Kenway, J, Kraack, A and Hickey-Moody, A 2006, *Masculinity beyond the metropolis*, Palgrave Macmillan, Basingstoke.

Kitzinger, C and Kitzinger, J 2015, 'How to plan for a good death', *Guardian*, 19 June, www.theguardian.com/lifeandstyle/2015/jun/19/how-to-plan-for-a-good-death-sheila-kitzinger?CMP=share_btn_fb accessed 7 July 2015.

Langer, L 1991, *Holocaust testimonies: the ruins of memory*, Yale University Press, Newhaven CT.

Lash, S 1994, 'Reflexivity and its doubles: structure, aesthetics, community', in U Beck, A Giddens and S Lash, *Reflexive modernisation*, Polity Press, Cambridge.

Latour, B 2007, *Reassembling the social: an introduction to actor-network theory*, Oxford University Press, Oxford.

Law, J 2004, *After method: mess in social science research*, Routledge, London and New York.

Leventhal, R S (ed.) 1994, *Reading after Foucault: institutions, disciplines, and technologies of the self in Germany, 1750–1830*, Wayne State University Press, Detroit MI.

Luhmann, N 1993, *Risk: a sociological theory*, Aldine de Gruyter, New York.

Lupton, D 1995, *The imperative of health: public health and the regulated body*, Sage, London and Thousand Oaks CA.

Lupton, D 1998, *The emotional self: a sociocultural exploration*, Sage, London.

Lupton, D 1999a, *Risk*, Routledge, London and New York.

Lupton, D 1999b, 'Monsters in metal cocoons: "road rage" and cyborg bodies', *Body and Society*, vol. 5, no. 1, pp. 57–72.

Lupton, D and Petersen, A 1996, *The new public health: health and self in the age of risk*, Sage, London.

Lupton, D and Tulloch, J 1998, 'The adolescent "unfinished body", reflexivity and HIV/AIDS risk', *Body and Society*, vol. 4, no. 2, pp. 19–34.

Lyon, M 2009, 'Emotion, embodiment and agency: the place of a social emotions perspective in the cross-disciplinary understanding of emotional processes', in B Rottger-Rossler and H J Markowitsch (eds), *Emotions as bio-cultural processes*, Springer, New York.

Machin, M A and Sankey, K S 2008, 'Relationships between young drivers' personality characteristics, risk perceptions, and driving behaviour', *Accident Analysis and Prevention*, vol. 40, pp. 541–547.

MacIntyre, A 1981, *After virtue: a study in moral theory*, Duckworth, London.

Mackenzie, O 2003, *Enhancing the safety of young drivers*, Roads Corporation, Kew, Victoria.

McAdams, D P 1996, *The stories we live by: personal myths and the making of the self*, Guilford Press, New York.

McDonald, R 2008, 'Grace and surrender: surfing and the fascist aesthetic', *Times Literary Supplement*, 16 May, p. 19.

McKnight, A J and McKnight, A S 2003, 'Young novice drivers: careless or clueless?' *Accident Analysis and Prevention*, vol. 35, no. 6, pp. 921–925.

McQueen, D V and Kickbusch, I 2007, 'Introduction: health promotion the origins of the third public health revolution leading to a new public health', in D V McQueen and I Kickbusch, *Health and modernity: the role of theory in health promotion*, Springer, New York.

Males, M 2005, 'California's graduated driver license law: effect on teenage drivers' deaths through 2005', *Journal of Safety Research*, vol. 38, no. 6, pp. 651–659.

Males, M 2006, 'Teen drivers: what are the real risks?' viewed 11 August 2011, http://homeearthlinknet/~mmales/

Males, M 2009, 'Poverty as a determinant of young drivers' fatal crash risks', *Journal of Safety Research*, vol. 40, no. 6, pp. 443–448.

Malik, K 2000, *Man, beast and zombie: what science can and cannot tell us about human nature*, Weidenfeld and Nicholson, London.

Mallick, J, Johnston, J, Goren, N and Kennedy, V 2007, *Drugs and driving in Australia: a survey of community attitudes, experience and understanding*, Australian Drug Foundation, Melbourne.

Marinetti, F 1909/1972, 'The founding and manifesto of Futurism', in R W Flint (ed.), *Marinetti: selected writings edited*, Secker and Warburg, London.

Marinetti, F 1916/1972, 'The new religion-morality of speed', in R W Flint (ed.), *Marinetti: selected writings*, Secker and Warburg, London.

Maunders, D and Sangster, J 1995, *Youth work with high risk young drivers*, RMIT University, Melbourne.

Mayhew, D R 2007, 'Driver education and graduated licensing in North America: past, present, and future', *Journal of Safety Research*, vol. 38, no. 2, pp. 229–235.

Mayhew, D R, Simpson, H M and Pak, A 2002, 'Changes in collision rates among novice drivers during the first months of driving', *Accident Analysis and Prevention*, vol. 35, no. 5, pp. 683–691.

Merleau-Ponty, M 2008, *Phenomenology of perception*, Routledge, London and New York.

Metropolitan Fire and Emergency Services Board, Community Education Department 2006, *Fit To Drive half day workshop road crash case study: Monavale Road*, MFB, Melbourne.

Midgley, M 1994, *The ethical primate: humans, freedom and morality*, Routledge, London.

Midgley, M 2001, *Science and poetry*, Routledge, London and New York.

Midgley, M 2003, *Heart and mind: the varieties of moral experience*, Routledge, London and New York.

Midgley, M 2006, *Science and poetry*, Routledge, London and New York.

Millstein, S and Halpern-Felsher, B 2002, 'Perceptions of risk and vulnerability', *Journal of Adolescent Health*, vol. 31, no. 1, Supplement 1, pp. 10–27.

Mitchell, W, Bunton, R and Green, E (eds) 2004, *Young people, risk and leisure: constructing identities in everyday life*, Palgrave Macmillan, Basingstoke.

Mol, A and Law, J 2006, 'Complexities: an introduction', in *Complexities: social studies of knowledge practices*, Duke University Press, Durham NC.

Montelle, Y-P 2009, *Paleoperformance: the emergence of theatricality as social practice*, University of Chicago Press, Chicago.

Montero, K, Rowland, B, Maunders, D and Kelly, L 2002, *Reducing the toll*, VicRoads, Melbourne.

Montero, K, Sangster, J and Maunders, D 1997, *Survival on the roads: a program to develop safer young drivers and passengers*, RMIT Centre for Youth Affairs Research and Development/VicRoads, Melbourne.

Montero, K and Spencer, G 2009, 'Fit to Drive: an innovative peer education approach to road safety in schools', presented at the First Asia-Pacific Conference on Health Promotion and Education, 18–19 July, Chiba City, Japan.

Montero, K, Spencer, G and Ariens, B 2009, 'Smartroads: training Indonesian workers to become road safety ambassadors in industrial and community settings', *Global Health Promotion*, vol. 19, pp. 19–26.

Mooney, C G 2000, *Theories of childhood: an introduction to Dewey, Montessori, Erickson, Piaget and Vygotsk*, Redleaf Press, St Paul MN.

Mukherjee, N 2008, 'The only way is down after ultimate high: Tim Winton book review' (published date: 25 May), *Scotland on Sunday*, accessed 8 July 2008, http://scotlandonsunday.scotsman.com/bookreviews/The-only-way-is-down.4116836.jp

Muuss, R E 1996, *Theories of adolescence*, 6th edn, McGraw-Hill, New York.

Nagel, T 1986, *The view from nowhere*, Oxford University Press, New York.

Nation, M, Crusto, C, Wandersman, A, Kumpfer, K, Seybolt, D, Morrisey-Kane, E and Davino, K 2003, 'What works in prevention: principles of effective prevention programs', *American Psychologist*, June/July.

Noe, A 2009, *Out of our heads*, Hill and Wang, New York.

Nussbaum, M C 2001a, *The fragility of goodness: luck and ethics in Greek tragedy and philosophy*, Cambridge University Press, Cambridge and New York.

Nussbaum, M C 2001b, *Upheavals of thought: the intelligence of emotions*, Cambridge University Press, Cambridge and New York.

Ochs, E and Capps, F 2001, *Living narrative: creating lives in everyday storytelling*, Harvard University Press, Cambridge MA.

O'Neill, E 2010, 'A work in progress: the adolescent brain', *The University of Melbourne Voice*, vol. 6, no. 3, March-April.

Patel, R 2010, 'Creativity and partnership', in J Batsleer and B Davies (eds), *What is youth work?*, Learning Matters, Exeter.

Paterson, M 2007, *Automobile politics, ecology and cultural political economy*, Cambridge University Press, Cambridge.

Patience, A 1992, 'The hard culture', in R Kosky, H D Eshkevari and G Kneebone (eds), *Breaking out: challenges in adolescent mental health in Australia*, Australian Government Publishing Service, Canberra.

Payne, M 2005, 'Working with groups', in R Harrison and C Wise (eds), *Working with young people*, Sage, London.

Peden, M, Oyegbite, K, Ozanne-Smith, J, Hyder, A, Branche, C, Rahman, F, Rivara, F and Bartolmeos, K 2008, *World report on child injury prevention*, World Health Organisation, Geneva.

Peden, M, Scurfield, R, Sleet, D, Mohan, D, Hyder, A A, Jarawan, E and Mathers, C (eds) 2004, *The world report on road traffic injury prevention*, World Health Organisation, Geneva.

Pike, J and Colquhoun, D 2010, 'Embodied childhood in the health promoting school', in R Colls and K Colquhoun Hurschelmann (eds), *Contested bodies of childhood and youth*, Palgrave Macmillan, Basingstoke.

Pike, J and Kelly, P 2014, *The moral geographies of children, young people and food: beyond Jamie's school dinners*, Palgrave, London.

Plant, M 1992, *Risk-takers: alcohol, drugs, sex and youth*, Tavistock/Routledge, London and New York.

Polanyi, M 1983, *The tacit dimension*, Peter Smith, Gloucester MA.

Polkinghorne, D E 1988, *Narrative knowing and the human sciences*, State University of New York Press, Albany.

Polkinghorne, D E 1991, 'Narrative and self-concept', *Journal of Narrative and Life History*, vol. 1, nos. 2 and 3, pp. 135–153.

Poynting, S and White, R 2004, 'Challenging the soft cop syndrome', *Youth Studies Australia*, vol. 23, no. 4, pp. 39–45.

Preusser, D 2003, 'Young driver crash risk', *Annual proceedings, Association for the Advancement of Automotive Medicine*, vol. 47, pp. 527–532.

Probyn, E 2010, 'How do children taste? Young people and the production and consumption of food', in K Hőrschelmann and R Colls (eds), *Contested bodies of childhood and youth*, Palgrave Macmillan, London.

RACV/VicHealth 2005, *Common solutions*, VicHealth, Melbourne.

Reyna, V and Farley, F 2007, 'Is the teen brain too rational?', *Scientific American Mind*, vol. 17, no. 6, pp. 58–65.

Richardson, L 1998, 'Writing: a method of inquiry', in N K Denzin and Y S Lincoln (eds), *Collecting and interpreting qualitative materials*, Sage, Thousand Oaks CA.

Richardson, L 2000, 'Writing: a method of inquiry', in N K Denzin and Y S Lincoln (eds), *Handbook of qualitative research* (2nd edn, pp. 923–948), Sage, Thousand Oaks CA.

Richardson, R (ed.) 2010, 'Introduction: opening an eye of the world', in W James, *The heart of William James: edited and with an introduction by Robert Richardson*, Harvard University Press, Cambridge MA.

Rimmon-Kenan, S 1983, *Narrative fiction: contemporary poetics*, Methuen, London.

Roberts, S 2010, 'One step forward, one step Beck: a contribution to the ongoing conceptual debate in youth studies', *Journal of Youth Studies*, vol. 15, no. 3, pp. 389–401.

Rose, N 1996, 'Psychiatry as a political science: advanced liberalism and the administration of risk', *History of the Human Sciences*, vol. 9, no. 2, pp. 1–23.

Rose, N 1999, *Powers of freedom: reframing political thought*, Cambridge University Press, Cambridge.

Rose, S 2005, *The future of the brain: the promise and perils of tomorrow's neuroscience*, Oxford University Press, New York.

Rowe, F, Stewart, D and Patterson, C 2007, 'Promoting school connectedness through whole school approaches', *Health Education*, vol. 107, no. 6, pp. 524–542.

Rozik, E 2002, *The roots of theatre: rethinking ritual and other theories of origin*, University of Iowa Press, Iowa City.

Russell, M 2006, 'Rev heads', *The Age*, 18 June.

Sabbagh, L 2006, 'The teen brain, hard at work', *Scientific American Mind*, vol. 17, no. 4, pp. 20–25.

Scheper-Hughes, N and Lock, M 1987, 'The mindful body: a prolegomenon to future work in medical anthropology', *Medical Anthropology Quarterly*, vol. 1, pp. 6–41.

Scheub, H 1998, *Story*, University of Wisconsin Press, Madison.

Scott, S and Williams, G 1992, 'Introduction', in S Scott, G Williams, S Platt and H Thames (eds), *Private risks and public danger*, Avebury, Aldershot.

Scott-Parker, B, Watson, B and King, M J 2009, 'Understanding the psychosocial factors influencing the risky behaviour of young drivers', *Transportation Research Part F*, vol. 12, pp. 470–482.

Senserrick, T M 2007, 'Recent developments in young driver education, training and licensing in Australia', *Journal of Safety Research*, vol. 38, pp. 237–244.

Senserrick, T and Haworth, N 2004, 'Young driver research: where are we now? What do we still need to know?' 2004 Road Safety Research, Policing and Education Conference, Perth, Australia, 14–16 November.

Sercombe, H 2010, 'The "teen brain" research: critical perspectives', *Youth and Policy*, vol. 105, November, pp. 71–80.

Sheehan, M, Cahill, H, Rowling, L, Marshall, B, Wyn, J and Holdsworth, R 2002, 'Establishing a role for schools in mental health promotion: the MindMatters project', in L Rowling, G Martin and L Walker (eds), *Mental health promotion and young people: concepts and practice*, McGraw-Hill, Sydney.

Shope, J T 2007, 'Graduated driver licensing: review of results since 2002', *Journal of Safety Research*, vol. 38, pp. 165–175.

Shope, J T, Waller, P F, Raghunathan, T E and Patil, S M 2001, 'Adolescent antecedents of high-risk driving behavior into young adulthood: substance use and parental influences', *Accident Analysis and Prevention*, vol. 33, no. 5, pp. 649–658.

Smith, M 1988, *Developing youth work: informal education, mutual aid and popular practice*, Open University Press, Milton Keynes and Philadelphia PA.

Spence, J, Devanney, C and Noonan, K 2006, *Youth work: voices of practice*, research report by Durham University and Weston Spirit, National Youth Agency, Leicester.

Spencer, G and Montero, K 2011, 'Empowering youth in schools to be safer road users: peer-led by undergraduates', Australian Council of Road Safety Conference, September, Melbourne.

Spencer, G, Montero, K and Rowland, B 2006, *Fit To Drive: a program to enhance the safety of young drivers*, Unpublished report, Melbourne.

Spinosa, C, Flores, F and Dreyfus, H L 1997, *Disclosing new worlds: entrepreneurship, democratic action, and the cultivation of solidarity*, MIT Press, Cambridge MA.

Spruijt-Metz, D 1999, *Adolescence, affect and health*, Psychology Press, Hove.

Steinberg, L 2005, 'Cognitive and affective development in adolescence', *Trends in Cognitive Science*, vol. 9, no. 2, pp. 68–75.

Steinberg, L 2008, 'A social neuroscience perspective on adolescent risk-taking', *Developmental Review*, vol. 28, pp. 78–106.

Styles, T, Imberger, K and Catchpole, J 2005, *Understanding risk-taking by young male drivers*, research report ARR 363, ARRB Group, Vermont South, Victoria.

Sunstein, C R 2008, 'Adolescent risk-taking and social meaning: a commentary', *Developmental Review*, vol. 28, pp. 145–152.

Szego, J 2010, 'The need for speed', *The Age*, 21 January.

Tait, G 1995, 'Shaping the "at-risk youth": risk, governmentality and the Finn Report', *Discourse*, vol. 16, no. 1, pp. 123–134.

Tait, G 2000, *Youth, sex and government*, Peter Lang, New York.

Tati, J 2008, *Trafic*, Criterion Collection, Chicago.

Taylor-Gooby, P and Zinn, J O 2006, 'Current directions in risk research: new developments in psychology and sociology', *Risk Analysis*, vol. 26, no. 2, pp. 397–411.

Theweleit, K 1996, *Male fantasies volume 2: male bodies: psychoanalysing the white terror*, University of Minnesota Press, Minneapolis.

Threadgold, S 2011, 'Should I pitch my tent in the middle ground? On "middling tendency", Beck and inequality in youth sociology', *Journal of Youth Studies*, vol. 14, no. 4, pp. 381–393.

Todres, L 2007, *Embodied enquiry: phenomenological touchstones for research, psychotherapy and spirituality*, Palgrave Macmillan, Basingstoke.

Toroyan, T and Peden, M (eds) 2007, *Youth and road safety*, World Health Organisation, Geneva.

Transport Accident Commission 2012, 'TAC road safety statistical summary', viewed 18 October 2012, www.tacsafety.com.au/jsp/statistics/roadtollannualdo?areaID=12 andtierID=1andnavID=17

Transport Accident Commission 2015, www.tac.vic.gov.au/road-safety/schools/school-resources/steve-biddulph

Truby, J 2007, *The anatomy of story: 22 steps to becoming a master storyteller*, Faber and Faber, New York.

Tulloch, J and Lupton, D 2003, *Risk and everyday life*, Sage, London.

United Nations 2011, 'United Nations Decade of Action for Road Safety 2011–2020', viewed 25 October 2012, www.un.org/en/roadsafety/

Urry, J 2007, *Mobilities*, Polity Press, Cambridge.

Vassallo, S, Smart, D, Cockfield, S, Guatillake, T, Harris, A and Harrison, W 2010, *In the driver's seat II: beyond the early driving years (research report no. 17)*, Australian Institute of Family Studies, Melbourne.

Vassallo, S, Smart, D, Sanson, A, Harrison, W, Harris, A, Cockfield, S and McIntyre, A 2007, 'Risky driving among young Australian drivers: trends, precursors and correlates', *Accident Analysis and Prevention*, vol. 39, pp. 444–458.

Vick, M 2003, 'Danger on the roads! Masculinity, the car, and safety', *Youth Studies Australia*, vol. 22, no. 1, pp. 32–37.

Vick, M 2005, '"I am a good driver": young people's construction of themselves as road users', *Youth Studies Australia*, vol. 24, no. 4, pp. 28–34.

VicRoads 2005, 'Young driver safety and graduated licensing discussion paper', VicRoads, Melbourne.

VicRoads 2006, *Kids on the move: traffic safety education for primary schools*, VicRoads, Kew, Victoria.

Victorian Government Department of Human Services 2008, 'Vulnerable youth framework discussion paper', Melbourne, Victoria.

Walker, L 1999, 'Hydraulic sexuality and hegemonic masculinity: young working-class men and car culture', in R White (ed.), *Australian youth subcultures: on the margins and in the mainstream*, Australian Clearinghouse for Youth Studies, Hobart.

Weick, K E 1995, *Sensemaking in organizations*, Sage, Thousand Oaks CA.

Weiss, J 2006, 'The teen driver', *Pediatrics*, vol. 118, no. 6, pp. 2570–2581, doi: 10.1542/peds.2006-2830.

Whelan, M and Oxley, J 2007, *Going solo: a resource for parents of P-plate drivers*, Monash University Accident Research Centre (MUARC), Clayton, Victoria.

White, H 1980, 'The value of narrativity in the representation of reality', *Critical Inquiry*, vol. 7, no. 1, 'On narrative', pp. 5–27, University of Chicago Press, Chicago.

Williams, A F 2003, 'Teenage drivers: patterns of risk', *Journal of Safety Research*, vol. 34, no. 1, pp. 5–15.

Winton, T 2008, *Breath*, Picador, London.

Wood, J 2008, *How fiction works*, Jonathan Cape, London.

Woodman, D 2009, 'The mysterious case of the pervasive choice biography', *Journal of Youth Studies*, vol. 12, no. 3, pp. 243–256.

World Health Organisation 2010, 'What is a health promoting school?' viewed 24 November 2010, www.whoint/school_youth_health/gshi/hps/en/indexhtml

Young, K 2006, *The art of youth work*, Russell House, Lyme Regis.

Youth Policy Development Council (YPDC) 1987, *Health for youth – final report: policy and strategies*, YPDC, Melbourne.

Youthsafe 2006, 'Adolescent development and risk taking', *Youthsafe Newsletter*, Spring.

Ziguras, C 2004, *Self-care: embodiment, personal autonomy and the shaping of health consciousness*, Routledge, London.

Zinn, J O 2009, *Social theories of risk and uncertainty: an introduction*, Blackwell, Malden MA.

Index

absence as Otherness *see* Law, John; storytelling in health promotion
acting (Rozik) 32
adolescent brain development and risk 55–6; *see also* choosing agents, young people as
Aesop's fables *see* chaos and control (Greek tragedy)
After Method (Law) 1
agency *see* choosing agents, young people as
alienation effect (Brecht) 74
Anything? (film) 112, 113
Apollonian/Dionysian dichotomy *see* chaos and control (Greek tragedy)
Aristotle 17, 129, 134–5
audience as decoder of intention (Montelle) 32–3
Australia: Department of Education and Early Childhood Development (DEECD) Traffic Safety Education Unit xiii; Education Department xiii; Graduated Licensing System 5, 6
'avoiding a bad' (James) 38, 39

backshadowing 110–11
Bakhtin, M. 115
Barnes, Julian 176–7
Barthes, Roland 121
Bauman, Zygmunt 72–3, 169, 170
Beck, Ulrich 51, 165, 166
behaviour change theory 4
Benjamin, Walter 58
Bernstein, Michael 112
Bessant, Judith 72
Biddulph, S. 56
Birthday (film) 103, 105–7, 109–10
blue river of truth (Wood) 62, 104–5
Boal, Augusto 162
bodily knowledge (Gendlin) 89
body and language *see* group work and meaning making
Bolton, R. 80
bounded agency (Evans) 165–6
Bourdieu, Pierre 11, 71, 101, 165
Braidotti, Rosi 141–3
Breath (Winton) 41–4, 60–2, 110–12, 172, 175
Brecht, Bertolt 68, 74–7
Brecht and the 'Theatre of Emotions' (interlude) 74–7
Brook, Peter 30
Buytendijk, F.J.J. 82

Capps, Lisa *see* Ochs and Capps
car culture *see* human-car-machine assemblage (interlude)
Carr-Gregg, Michael 56
Castel, Robert 145–8
chaos and control (Greek tragedy) 17, 125–44; fear and pity and Monavale story as tragedy 131–6; Kerry's story: Aeschylus or Aesop? (interlude) 130–1; the Monavale tragedy 125–30; the tragic and the problem of death 138–44; workshops, excerpts from 125–31, 136–8
choosing agents, young people as 17, 145–70; beyond agency in health promotion 163–70; dangerousness of risk 145–9; enactment of safe choices 155–63; FBC (Feelings, Behaviours, Consequences) formula 159–61; talking about/rating risks 149–55; workshops, excerpts from 148–63
Coffey, Julia 170
Collins, R 82–3

community of interest *see* storytelling in health promotion
Country Fire Authority (CFA) 33–4
crisis of reason (Grosz) 7

Damasio, Antonio 69, 78
dangerousness of risk *see* choosing agents, young people as
death, problem of *see* chaos and control (Greek tragedy)
death and devastation as allegory 171–9
Deleuze, Gilles 2
Department of Education and Early Childhood Development (DEECD) 33–4
dialogue as dangerous (Boal) 162
Dutta, Shomit 134

Ellos, William 121
embodied meaning making *see* group work and meaning making
emotions, values, and mobilising rationality 15–16, 64–84; Brecht and the 'Theatre of Emotions' (interlude) 74–7; Fridays with Graham, November 2009/Talking about feelings, behaviours, consequences (interlude) 79–81; health education, youth work and values 69–74; health promotion and emotion as embodied sociality 81–4; a moment of emotional truth 64–8; rediscovering emotions 77–9; workshops, excerpts from 64–8
Evans, Karen 165–6
existentialism 78–9

Farrugia, David 170
fascist psyche (Theweleit) 58–9
Fate/Reason dichotomy *see* chaos and control (Greek tragedy)
FBC (Feelings, Behaviours, Consequences) formula 159–61
fear and pity (Aristotle) 134
Fit to Drive program: and embodied health promotion 8–12; facilitator training 90–5, 100, 118; Local Area Coordinators (LACs) 25, 35–6; origins of xii–xvi; Reducing the Toll program 70; student role models 34; as whole school curriculum approach 24–5; workshops, excerpts from 9–10, 20–3, 44–6, 64–8, 125–31, 136–8, 148–63; *see alsoindividual analyses*
Flanagan, Richard 85–6, 88, 163
Forster, E.M. 76–7
Foucault, Michel 72–3, 170; on governmentality 26, 55; limit experiences 3, 23, 175; technologies and practice of the self 169
Frankston-Mornington Peninsula Young Driver Safety committee xiii
Fridays with Graham, November 2009/Talking about feelings, behaviours, consequences (interlude) 79–81
Futurist movement *see* human-car-machine assemblage (interlude)

Gadamer, H.-G. 95, 96, 97, 98, 162
gathering (Law) 178
Gendlin, Eugene 13, 89, 98, 99–100
Giddens, Anthony 51, 52
Goffman, Erving 30–1
the 'good' (James) 14, 23, 38–9
good death/tragic death *see* chaos and control (Greek tragedy)
Greek tragedy analogy *see* chaos and control (Greek tragedy)
Grosz, Elizabeth 6, 7
group work and meaning making 16, 85–102; body and language 98–102; does her body think? (Flanagan) 85–6, 88; embodied meaning making 87–90; facilitator training 90–5, 100; group agreement and socialisation 95–8; group session, excerpt from 90–3

habitus (Bourdieu) 71
Haraway, Donna 8, 141, 171
hard culture (Patience) 59
Hayles, Katherine 141
Hayman, Suzie 138
health education literature 71
health sciences and risk behaviours 54
Herbrechter, Stefan 141–2
Hille, David 45, 46, 104
human-car-machine assemblage (interlude) 56–60
Hume, David 75
Hunter, Ian 23, 26–7, 164, 169
Husserl, Edmund 97, 120

inexperienced drivers *see* rationality and risk, limits and possibilities
intentional space (Brook) 30
Interludes: the aesthetics and erotics of the human-car-machine assemblage 56–60; Brecht and the 'Theatre of Emotions' 74–7; Fridays with

Graham, November 2009/Talking about feelings, behaviours, consequences 79–81; Kerry's story xii–xvi, 118–19, 130–1, 178–9
interrelated multiplicity (Todres) 13
'irreal' spaces of schools *see* school based health promotion as complex assemblage

James, William 89; 'the Good' 14, 23, 38–9 *see also* school based health promotion as complex assemblage
Jarvis, Peter 73, 78–9, 81
Jim O'Brien's Story 107–8, 123
Johnson, Mark 69, 78, 88–9, 99, 100–1
Journal of Youth Studies 165–6
journey as narrative quest *see* storytelling in health promotion
Julie's Story 103–4, 109–10, 121
Jünger, Ernst 57

Katz, Jack 69
Kelly, Peter (references)
Kitzinger, Celia 139
Kitzinger, Jenny 139
Kitzinger, Sheila 138–9
knowing as situated inquiry 2

Langer, Susanne 31, 116
language *see* choosing agents, young people as; group work and meaning making
Lash, Scott 54–5
Latour, Bruno 2, 167–8, 170
Law, John: absence as Otherness 3; account of 1999 train collision as allegory 171–4; *After Method* 1–2; concept of gathering 178; and Haraway's embodied knowledges 8; on limits of natural science in study of human behavior 7; on method assemblage 2–3, 12, 14, 61, 102; ontological politics 173–4
lived body (Todres) 87
Lovett, William 27
Lupton, Deborah 49–50, 54, 75–6, 78
Lyon, Margaret 82

MacIntyre, Alasdair 36–7, 121, 123
Malik, Kenan 96
Marinetti, Filippo 57, 58
meaning making *see* group work and meaning making
Merleau-Ponty, M. 88
method assemblage (Law) 2–3, 12, 14, 61, 102, 173–4; *see also* school based health promotion as complex assemblage
Metropolitan Fire Brigade (MFB) 33–4, 35, 125–31
Midgley, Mary 6, 7, 69, 76, 77
Mills, C. Wright 62
Mitchell, W. 52
Mol, Annemarie 1
Montelle, Y.-P. 30–1
Montero, Kerry (references)
moral emotions *see* emotions, values, and mobilising rationality
moral project of schooling 26–7; *see also* school based health promotion as complex assemblage; storytelling in health promotion
Mothers Against Drink Driving (MADD) 119
myth as narrative (Ellos) 121

narrative devices *see* storytelling in health promotion
The Narrow Road to the Deep North (Flanagan) 163
Nietzsche 57
Youthsafe Newsletter 56
Nussbaum, Martha 69, 77–8

Ochs and Capps 110, 111, 112, 114–15, 122
Ochs, Eleanor *see* Ochs and Capps
ontological politics (Law) 173–4

A Passage to India (Forster) 76–7
Patience, Allan 59
People Skills (Bolton) 80
police departments: role of Youth Resource Officers (YROs) 25
Polkinghorne, Donald E. 114
The Posthuman (Braidotti) 141–3
Powers of Freedom (Rose) 26
The Presentation of Self in Everyday Life (Goffman) 30
preventive strategies of social administration (Castel) 145–8

RACV/VicHealth Common Solutions project 11–12, 33–4
rating the risk *see* choosing agents, young people as
rationality and risk, limits and possibilities 14–15, 41–63; the aesthetics and erotics of the

human-car-machine assemblage (interlude) 56–60; beyond rationality and risk 60–2; *Breath* and the horror of the mundane (Winton) 41–4, 60–2; cold, hard facts 44–7; risk, meanings of (Lupton) 49–50; workshops, excerpts from 44–6; young people, road safety and risk 47–52; young people and problem of risk 52–60
Reassembling the Social (Latour) 167
recognisable characters (MacIntyre) 36–7
Reducing the Toll program xiii
rethinking the school *see* school based health promotion as complex assemblage
Rethinking the School (Hunter) 26–7
retrospective knowing *see* storytelling in health promotion
Richardson, Robert 39
Ricoeur, Paul 114
risk, meanings of (Lupton) 49–50
at-risk concept *see* rationality and risk, limits and possibilities
risk frameworks and social education 8
Risk Society (Beck) 51
risk taking *see* rationality and risk, limits and possibilities
ritual (Rozik) 32
road movie genre 123
road safety education: in Australia xii–xiii; as 'avoiding a bad' (James) 38; and moral concerns 122; in schools 8; *see alsoindividual programs*
road safety research 5–6, 48–9
road trauma statistics xii
Roberts, Steven 165–6, 168
Rose, Nikolas 11, 23, 26, 28, 29, 147, 148
Rowland-Ariens, Bern xii
Royal Automobile Club of Victoria (RACV) 11–12
Rozik, Eli 31–2

safe choices *see* choosing agents, young people as
Scheub, Harold 108, 116, 117
Schiller, Friedrich 129–30, 136
school based health promotion as complex assemblage 14, 20; and 'the Good' (James) 23; 'irreal' spaces of schools 24–9; and Law's method assemblage 23; mobilisation for 'the Good' 37–40; players in school based performance 33–7; workshop settings as theatre 29–33
schools as governable spaces *see* school based health promotion as complex assemblage
Scott, S. 52
second-wave cognitive science (Johnson) 88
The Sense of an Ending (Barnes) 176–7
Shakespeare 129–30, 136
Shannon's Story 105–10
shared vocabularies (Weick) 161–2
Shuttleworth, James Kay 27
sideshadowing *see* storytelling in health promotion
silence *see* group work and meaning making
Sleith, Shannon 106
social theory (Braidotti) 141–3
sociological imagination (Mills) 62
Spencer, Graham, role in Fit to Drive xii, 22–3, 30, 32, 34, 37, 64–8, 70, 79–81, 83, 96, 103–4, 106–7, 107, 118, 120, 123
Spinosa, C. 119
storytelling in health promotion 16–17, 34–5, 103–24; audience and narrative devices 108–13; backshadowing 110–11; characteristics of story and narrative 113–18; examples of 103; Graham's Story 107; Jim O'Brien's Story 107–8, 123; Julie's Story 103–4, 109–10, 121; Kerry's story: understanding Jim (interlude) 118–19; narrative quest and pursuit of the moral 121–4; Shannon's Story 105–10; sideshadowing 112–13; story, empathy and understanding 118–21
Survival on the Roads program xiii, 151–5

Tait, Gordon 147
Tati, Jacques 60
technologically amplified aestheticism (Benjamin) 58
Teenage Road Accident Group 33–4
teen brain theories *see* rationality and risk, limits and possibilities
teller–interlocutor relationship (Ochs and Capps) 115–16
theatre as imagistic medium (Rozik) 31–2
theatre as institution (Montelle) 30–1
'Theatre of Emotions' (Brecht) 74
theatricality as social practice (Goffman) 30–1

Theweleit, Klaus 58
Threadgold, Steven 165, 166, 168
Todres, Les 13, 87, 96, 97, 98, 119, 120
Trafic (film) 60
tragedy *see* chaos and control (Greek tragedy)
Transport Accident Commission (TAC) xii, 33–4, 56, 70, 112
Tulloch, J. 54

understanding-as-movement *see* group work and meaning making
United Nations (UN): Decade of Action for Road Safety 11

VicHealth 11–12
VicRoads xii–xiv, 49, 152; Young Driver Resource 70
Victoria, Australia: Arrive Alive strategy 33–4
Victoria Police Department: road safety education xiii; Youth Resource Officers (YROs) 33, 44–7
virtue ethics (Bessant) 72

Wanting (Flanagan) 85–6, 88
Weick, Karl 161–2
White, Hayden 116
Williams, G. 52
Winton, Tim 41–4, 60–2, 110–11, 172, 175
Wood, James 62, 104–5
Woodman, Dan 165–6, 168
workshop settings as theatre *see* school based health promotion as complex assemblage

young driver research 5–6
young people and health promotion, introduction 1–19; embodiment and aesthetics of meaning making 12–14; Fit to Drive program and embodied health promotion 8–12; health promotion as complex assemblage 1–7; Kerry's story 178–9; organization of book 14–19; summary conclusion 171–9

Zinn, J.O. 50–1